Beyond Words Publishing, Inc.
20827 N.W. Cornell Road, Suite 500
Hillsboro, Oregon 97124-9808
503-531-8700

Copyright © 2003 by Ronda Gates and Beverly Whipple

Information in Appendix E, "Questions to Ask Your Doctor," copyright © 2000 National Osteoporosis Foundation. Used with permission.

Managing Editor: Julie Steigerwaldt
Copy Editor: Jade Chan
Proofreader: David Abel
Cover Design: Michelle Farinella
Interior Design: Dorral Lukas
Illustrations: Anita Jones
Composition: William H. Brunson Typography Services

Printed in the United States of America
Distributed to the book trade by Publishers Group West

Library of Congress Cataloging-in-Publication Data
Gates, Ronda.
    Outwitting osteoporosis : the smart woman's guide to bone health /
Ronda Gates, Beverly Whipple.
        p. cm.
    Includes bibliographical references and index.
    ISBN 1-58270-099-0
    1. Osteoporosis in women—Popular works.   2. Osteoporosis—Popular
works.   I. Whipple, Beverly.   II. Title.
RC931.O73G377   2003
616.7'16—dc21

2003000979

The corporate mission of Beyond Words Publishing, Inc.:
Inspire to Integrity

OUTWITTING OSTEOPOROSIS

THE SMART WOMAN'S GUIDE TO BONE HEALTH

Also by Ronda Gates

The Lowfat Lifestyle with Valerie Parker

Nutrition Nuggets and More!/Changes: The Rest of the Story

Smart Eating: Choosing Wisely, Living Lean with Covert Bailey

The Scale Companion: How to Find Your Ideal Body Weight
with Frank Katch, Ph.D., and Victor Katch, Ph.D.

Beauty, More Than Skin Deep

LIFESTYLES PLANNER weight management software

Also by Beverly Whipple

The G Spot and Other Discoveries About Human Sexuality
with Alice Kahn Ladas, Ed.D., and John D. Perry, Ph.D.

Safe Encounters: How Women Can Say Yes to Pleasure and No to Unsafe Sex
with Gina Ogden, Ph.D.

OUTWITTING OSTEOPOROSIS

THE SMART WOMAN'S GUIDE TO BONE HEALTH

RONDA GATES, M.S.
BEVERLY WHIPPLE, PH.D.

BEYOND
WORDS
Publishing
I N C

To mothers and daughters everywhere.
—Ronda

To my grandchildren, Kayla, Travis, Valeria, William, and Elyse, with love.
—Beverly

Contents

Contents

Acknowledgments

No published book is created by its authors alone. In this case, friends took what we thought was a stellar project and returned it to us covered with red marks, suggestions for revised phrasing, and questions, such as "I don't know what this means," or "You already said this," or "A whole chapter could be developed on this topic." We discovered our egos could survive constructive criticism, sort through feedback, and accept suggestions that clarified everything we were trying to say. Each draft (and there were many) was better than the last.

We thank the people who made *Outwitting Osteoporosis* possible:

In Ronda's office, Sally Hedman, for her willingness to edit and compile resources.

In Beverly's office, Jim Whipple, for manning the computer when it wouldn't perform as expected; Sue Whipple-Forcier, R.N., M.S., for a younger woman's perspective; Pat Bessey, for a middle-aged woman's perspective; and Lois Ann Kastl and Vivian Heiler, for helping us remember what is important to women as they get older.

Dr. Robert Lindsay, our highly respected physician and friend, and the former president of the National Osteoporosis Foundation, for generously reading and editing our original text.

Acknowledgments

Dr. Eric Orwell of Oregon Health & Science University, who enlightened us about men's osteoporosis issues and reviewed the chapter on men.

Dr. Lana Holstein, author of *How to Have Magnificent Sex* and women's health director at Canyon Ranch Health Resorts, and Dr. Marisa Weiss, author of *Living Beyond Breast Cancer* and president of *www.breastcancer.org*, our friends and colleagues, whose perspectives, as women and physicians, assured that our content included practical advice for our readers.

Dianne Dunkelman, the awesome and energetic visionary, backbone, and founder of Speaking of Women's Health Foundation. The idea for this book was forged during a passionate discussion with Diane about women's health issues. She said, "Do bones first," and supported us through every page, providing feedback based on her experience with thousands of women whose lives she has touched.

Andi Miller for suggesting the title for this book.

Cynthia Black, Richard Cohn, Julie Steigerwaldt, and the rest of the Beyond Words staff who responded quickly to our calls and provided encouragement, patience, and support.

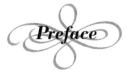

Preface

Once upon a time, the standard of health care for women was designed by and based on what we knew about men. Women were banned from drug trials. Scientists learned how men's bodies metabolized food, responded to exercise, and got sick and well. Then they extrapolated that information and applied it to women. Most physicians, pharmacists, and researchers were men. They told us how to take care of our bodies and, in most cases, we yielded to their authority. If women wanted to help people be well, we were relegated to roles as nursing assistants, research assistants, technologists, and health educators.

Thankfully, the face of women's health has changed. We have many more options than our mothers or grandmothers. Thanks to 1993 legislation, women must be included in all drug studies. When we seek medical care, we meet female physicians, nurse practitioners, and pharmacists. We've discovered we have options, so we ask questions, seek alternatives, and discuss these options with friends and families. Many of these new choices contribute to our ability to take control of our destinies and live a longer, more fulfilling, and healthier lives.

Sadly, not everyone has received the message. Compare the three following scenarios. Which of these women will you be?

Ruth

In 1993 Ruth was a vibrant eighty-year-old woman. She flourished in her role as a highly visible community leader, whose efforts to promote health education earned well-deserved accolades and a humanitarian award from the University of North Carolina Board of Directors.

One morning, just after her eightieth birthday, Ruth awakened with an all-too-familiar tightness in her chest. She used the bronchodilator prescribed for allergies and bronchospasms, took her thyroid medication and vitamins, ate breakfast, and went about her day. Later, she was paralyzed by a bronchospasm that literally "rattled her bones" when she coughed. When she finally caught her breath, she felt exhausted. Her back hurt. She decided the coughing spell had given her a muscle spasm, but she didn't let it stop her. Her stiffness increased and the discomfort in her back became more severe. By the next morning the slightest movement precipitated excruciating pain. A friend drove her to the hospital where X rays revealed that she had five spontaneous spinal fractures. Ruth was diagnosed with osteoporosis.

Ten years later, this ninety-year-old woman is seven inches shorter and has a dowager's hump. She uses a walker to prevent a fall. The last time she got in and out of a car she experienced three more painful spinal fractures, so she no longer leaves her home. Her mobility there is limited to walking from her bed, where she spends most of her time, to her kitchen table where, because her appetite has diminished, she eats only a few bites of the foods that satisfy her. She is in constant pain, which she alleviates with painkillers and muscle relaxants that impair her mental capabilities. She is scared. Most of her friends died long ago, so she is lonely. And she is angry. All these emotions are projected on the caretakers and family who have attempted to give her the support she needs.

Preface

Jean

Jean is Ruth's fifty-five-year-old daughter. She's learned her lesson well. After the wake-up call delivered by her mother's diagnosis, she decided to adopt an osteoporosis-preventing lifestyle. She joined and used a health club. She agreed to hormone replacement therapy despite concerns about its long-term use. She began taking a calcium supplement. So you can imagine her surprise when she received the results of her first bone density scan this year. It showed she has osteopenia, a loss of bone. In Jean's case, it's noticeable in her hip, pelvis, and shoulder. Although this news devastated her, her doctor wasn't so distressed. She cheered Jean's efforts and told her, "Your bone loss would probably have been worse if you'd been more sedentary. Keep up the good work." She added the good news that because there are new drug treatments to prevent bone loss, women no longer need to face the agony and pain caused by deteriorating bones. Jean shared her doctor's excitement when she learned there are exciting new drugs approved to treat osteoporosis. "Tell your women friends not to despair if they have been diagnosed with osteoporosis," her doctor said. "They should contact their doctors so they can learn how these miracle drugs that actually improve bone density and significantly decrease the risk of fracture can become part of a comprehensive treatment model." Jean agreed to spread the word.

Ann

Ann is Jean's twenty-eight-year-old daughter. She has been physically active all her life. She doesn't smoke or diet excessively. Her alcohol consumption is limited to an occasional glass of wine with dinner. She has heeded media information about good nutrition, takes a calcium with vitamin D supplement, and, since her grandmother's diagnosis, follows the guidelines for prevention of osteoporosis. Her bone density scan shows that her bones are strong for a woman her age. Since she is predisposed to osteoporosis, she plans to continue her active lifestyle. Unless there are unforeseen circumstances (a chronic illness, for example), she can expect to live a long life filled with the choices available to healthy, active, osteoporosis-free women.

WHAT YOU NEED TO KNOW

Osteoporosis is a condition that was not widespread until medical and technological advances for diagnosis and treatment of disease increased women's life spans. As they lived longer, more and more women developed osteoporosis. Here are alarming statistics every woman should know:

- Today, 45 percent of postmenopausal Caucasian women have osteoporosis.
- One in ten women over age sixty-five has a collapsed vertebra.
- Forty percent of all white women in the United States will sustain a hip fracture by age eighty if they fall.
- One-fifth of postmenopausal hip fracture patients die within one year of sustaining their injury.
- Sixty percent of patients who sustain a hip fracture never fully regain daily activity.

The good news is that women don't have to wait until they experience a fracture to discover that their bones are becoming more fragile. There are assessments that can predict risk and prompt early treatment. Best of all, a majority of the risk factors that predispose women to osteoporosis are lifestyle factors. Empowered with the knowledge and resources gained from this book, each of us can temper or prevent a disease state that leads to painful elderly years.

In order to make wise choices, women need accurate, useful, easy-to-understand information. We hope you will find what you need here.

—Ronda and Beverly

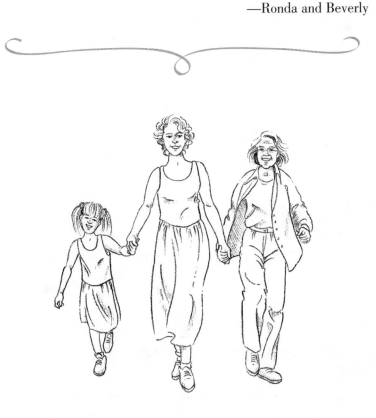

Section I

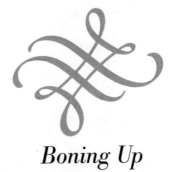

Boning Up

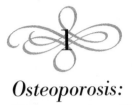

Osteoporosis:
A Life-Threatening Disease

Most women know aging brings an increased risk of declining health and multiple diseases. We have watched women friends and acquaintances and mothers age and die. We are used to hearing about deaths from heart disease, stroke, or cancer. But few of us are aware of another killer that steals more women's lives than breast cancer. It is osteoporosis, a bone disorder that predisposes bones to fractures.

Osteoporosis and a dowager's hump (curvature of the spine) used to be considered a natural part of life for an aging woman. That is no longer true. Today this common human bone disease is diagnosed in the old *and* in the young. Nevertheless, it is middle-aged women who are newly aware of osteoporosis as an important health issue. It is well described by its name: *Osteo* = bones and *Porosis* = porous. Osteoporosis literally means "porous bones."

Important Facts You Need to Know
In the United States:
- Osteoporosis is characterized by low bone mass and an increase in the risk of fracture.
- Women can lose up to 20 percent of bone mass after menopause.

- Osteoporosis threatens more than forty-four million Americans, 80 percent of whom are women.
- A study published in the *Journal of the American Medical Association* in December 2001, which screened the bone density of 200,000 healthy U.S. women age fifty or older, showed that almost 40 percent had undiagnosed osteopenia, and 7 percent had undiagnosed osteoporosis.
- Women with osteoporosis are four times more likely than healthy women to sustain a fracture in the next twelve months. Women with osteopenia are 1.8 times more likely to sustain a fracture in the next twelve months.
- Osteoporosis will cause a broken bone in one out of every two Caucasian women over age fifty. There is also significant risk, although it is lower, for non-Caucasian women (and for all men).
- Osteoporosis is the cause of more than 1.5 million spine, hip, wrist, and other fractures each year. These fractures affect one out of every six women.
- Costs for fractures from osteoporosis are in excess of $17 billion a year.
- If women in their thirties and forties don't take preventative action, it is estimated that by the year 2020 costs for osteoporosis-related fractures will be $60 billion annually.
- Unless prevention methods are adopted, it is projected that by 2020 there will be more than sixty million men and women over the age of fifty affected by this disease.

Women, Take Notice!

Unfortunately, most women don't find out they have osteoporosis until they fracture a bone, notice they have lost height, or develop curvature of the spine. One of the first symptoms may be back pain. That is why osteoporosis is called a "silent thief." It can progress without outward signs while, internally, potentially devastating consequences loom on the health horizon. Osteoporosis is a risk factor for fracture just as high blood pressure is a risk factor for stroke. Osteoporosis is like high blood pressure in another way: In most cases it can be prevented and treated with a combination of lifestyle, diet, and therapeutic approaches.

"Do Women Really Live Longer, or Do They Just Take Longer to Die?"

Today's healthy woman can expect to live eighty years. One of the consequences of living a long time is a decline in the body systems that function so optimally when we are young. One such system is the capacity to maintain bone density. Both men and women lose some bone mass as they age. People with osteoporosis lose an excessive amount of bone. The bone that is left is so porous, brittle, fragile, and weakened that it can snap under stresses that would not break a normal bone.

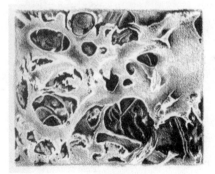
Normal Bone

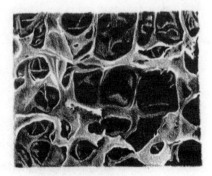
Osteoporotic Bone

If the bone that breaks is a hip bone, return to a previous level of activity is rare. Nearly one-third of women who break their hip are forced to move into long-term care facilities. Many die within six months. Fear, anxiety, and depression are common when women live with this disease. What woman would look forward to this lifestyle?

When doctors make the diagnosis of osteoporosis, they describe it as primary osteoporosis or secondary osteoporosis.

There are two types of primary osteoporosis:

Type I occurs as a result of the sudden drop in estrogen levels that occurs at menopause. This precipitates a decrease in bone mass that can set the stage for the hip, wrist, and forearm fractures that occur in a fall.

Type II occurs as a result of aging, when the osteoclastic activity that breaks down bone exceeds the osteoblastic activity that builds bones. This sets the stage for hip and spinal fractures that result in shortened height and a dowager's hump.

Secondary osteoporosis is precipitated by medications such as thyroid drugs and corticosteroids that treat other diseases. A child who uses steroid inhalers for asthma for many years might develop secondary osteoporosis.

When *You* Don't Have Osteoporosis

You don't have to be diagnosed with osteoporosis to be affected by the disease. Nearly three-quarters of the friends and relatives who provide care for osteoporosis patients are women, with 85 percent of these women over age forty-five. Described as "the sandwich generation" because they care for children *and* parents, these essential and overlooked caregivers have a critical role that will be compromised if they, too, fall victim to osteoporosis. That's the bad news.

There is also good news. Scientists have provided us with new knowledge of how bone mass increases, peaks, and declines. We can examine risk factors and use machines to measure the density of our bones. Researchers have eagerly embraced this information to explore new drug options for the prevention and treatment of osteoporosis. These developments can change the prognosis for family members and friends.

WHAT YOU NEED TO KNOW

By following the guidelines offered in this book, you can take charge of your life and your health. You can help prevent osteoporosis in yourself and in your daughters, and, as new drugs that reverse this disease emerge, help your mothers—even if they already have the disease.

Read on!

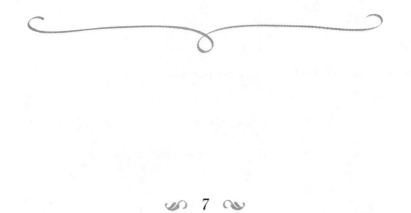

Why Women Are Different

Of course, women are different from men. It's obvious, and it's about more than physical appearance. Women think and communicate differently. Entire books have been written about the different speaking styles of men and women. Women are different on the inside, too. Their different reproductive organs produce different hormones, which have different functions. These differences play a big role in the diseases women might develop as they age. That's why researchers, doctors, and women who attend health conferences talk about "gender-specific biology."

Although both women and men get osteoporosis, the surging and receding hormones that accompany a woman's menstrual cycle contribute to the heightened risk, earlier onset, and overall prognosis of osteoporosis. But to discuss osteoporosis in women or men, we need some knowledge about how the human body functions.

Sex hormones are important for acquiring and maintaining bone mass in both women and men. Testosterone is the primary hormone for men, while estrogen is the primary hormone for women, although both men and women have testosterone and estrogen. These hormones escalate at puberty and subside as we age; however, estrogen declines faster and more abruptly in women than testosterone does in men. For women, the most apparent changes happen at the start of menstruation, during puberty, and when menopause begins in middle age.

How Menstruation Works

Most of the time our remarkable human body works using a complex feedback system, much in the same way that a thermostat responds to the temperature of your home. In a woman's reproductive, or sexual, system, her two reproductive organs—the ovaries—regulate the sexual thermostat. Each ovary contains structures called follicles, which hold egg cells. A woman is born with about 500,000 egg cells. By puberty, about seventy-five thousand are left. Only about four hundred to five hundred of these egg cells fully mature. The rest degenerate.

The female body also produces many hormones. Four of these—estrogen, progesterone, the follicle-stimulating hormone (FSH), and the luteinizing hormone (LH)—are the active hormones of a woman's menstrual cycle. Just after menstruation begins, when estrogen and progesterone levels are low, the hypothalamus—one of the action-oriented brain centers—starts to work. It stimulates the pituitary gland, which releases FSH and LH. The follicles, now stimulated by FSH and LH, produce the hormones estrogen and progesterone. This causes the lining of the uterus to thicken and become a potential source of nourishment for the development of one or more fertilized eggs. If male sperm does not fertilize the egg, the lining of the uterus breaks down, menstruation occurs, and the cycle begins again. Just as the thermostat turns on the heater in your home when it gets too cold, low levels of estrogen and progesterone begin the action of FSH and LH. High levels of estrogen and progesterone turn off that action.

Perimenopause and Menopause

Typically, a woman's transition into menopause is divided into three phases:

Perimenopause: The start of the transition—the time immediately prior to naturally occurring menopause—when the changes indicating the approach of menopause begin.

Menopause: The completion of the ovarian transition, marked by the last menstrual period. (Menopause is considered complete when a woman has not had a menstrual period for one year.)

Postmenopausal zest: The time when women tap into a new vitality.

The "change of life"—when estrogen levels decline significantly and the cyclical pattern of menstruation gradually stops—is a marker for women in many ways. Medically, the word "menopause" means the permanent end of menstruation. It is derived from the Greek words for "month" (*mensis*) and "cessation" (*pausis*). Menopause is a normal stage of a woman's life triggered by a decrease in estrogen levels. The transition can take as few as five or more than ten years. Even women as young as thirty-five experience perfectly normal physical and emotional symptoms of menopause. Perimenopause is the start of the transition, when women have fluctuating hormone levels and irregular ovulation.

The hormonal changes that take place during perimenopause and menopause are not unlike those that take place during puberty and pregnancy. There are pleasures but there may also be emotional swings. Smart women think of menopause as a period in their life when they are likely to be "hormonally challenged."

Until recently, we didn't know much about perimenopause. At the turn of the twentieth century, not many women lived past menopause. We didn't discuss it because it was an "embarrassing" subject and a life passage dreaded by many women. Menopause signaled aging, and people in the United States and in many other countries remain phobic about getting older. Even in our more enlightened times, as thousands of baby boomers move into this phase of life, there are still many myths and misconceptions about menopause. In a survey in which women were asked what was the worst part about this life passage, most said, "Not knowing what to expect is frightening."

Just as each woman experiences puberty and pregnancy differently, each goes through perimenopause and menopause in her own way. We have different levels of hormones circulating in our bodies and different diet patterns, exercise patterns, and life experiences. All of these factors affect our physiology. That is why the menopause experience can range from virtually no symptoms, except for the cessation of menstrual periods, to long-lasting symptoms, which can severely interfere with day-to-day living. Most of these reactions are prompted by three factors:

1. The level of circulating hormones
2. The intensity of hormonal changes
3. A woman's sensitivity to her hormonal changes

Ten to 15 percent of women breeze through this time with no discomfort, while another 10 to 15 percent experience severe symptoms. The majority of women (75 to 80 percent) have one or more perimenopausal symptoms that are inconvenient but manageable. (Even though we call them "symptoms," it is important to remember that menopause is not a disease but a normal phase of life.)

Symptoms of perimenopause and menopause that some women experience include:

Breast tenderness	Lack of sexual desire
Fatigue	Memory loss
Frequent urination	Mental sluggishness
Headaches	Moodiness
Heart palpitations	Night awakenings
Hot flashes	Night sweats
Insomnia	Pain with intercourse
Irregular periods	Unusual skin sensitivities
Irritability	Vaginal dryness
Joint pains	

It is unlikely that every woman will experience all these symptoms. That's the good news. The bad news is none of them are a welcome intrusion into daily life.

Smart women overcome the experiences that accompany menopause with a positive attitude. Hot flashes become "power surges," vaginal dryness becomes an "Astroglide opportunity," and memory loss becomes a "senior moment." A positive attitude can change everything.

It's All About Hormones

In a woman's mid-thirties, the ovarian production of hormones begins to decline. This process accelerates as a woman reaches her mid- to late-forties, when hormone levels fluctuate even more, causing irregular cycles and heavy bleeding. Estrogen is still produced in small amounts by the ovaries. Another form of estrogen, estrone, is produced in fat cells. Interestingly, heavy women whose weight predisposes them to other diseases experience fewer symptoms of perimenopause and menopause.

> More fat cells = more estrone = fewer symptoms of menopause

As a woman approaches menopause, her levels of estrogen and progesterone begin to drop, her supply of eggs dwindles, and the follicles lose their ability to respond to the FSH and LH stimulation. FSH and LH levels increase in an effort to make the ovaries produce more estrogen and progesterone.

Lower levels of estrogen and/or progesterone can result in periods of moodiness and depression. One reason is that the ovarian hormones interact with endorphins, biochemical substances in the brain that act like "internal morphine." Endorphins can block feelings of pain and give women a sense of well-being.

When women have both ovaries surgically removed, they experience an abrupt menopause. This surgery, known as a bilateral ovariectomy (or bilateral oophorectomy), often occurs at an earlier age than naturally occurring menopause. Women who undergo surgical menopause may be hit harder by the symptoms of menopause than women who move to this stage as a natural process of life. Women who have chemotherapy or radiation to their pelvic area to treat cancer can also experience premature ovarian failure. Also, 10 percent of women fall outside the expected norms for menopause and stop menstruating before their fortieth birthday.

Menopause Signals Bone Loss

As menopause begins and estrogen levels start to decline, women are more susceptible to bone loss. Estrogen deficiency is clearly associated with osteoporosis. Normally, estrogens bind to bone-forming osteoblasts, causing a chemical secretion that prevents osteoclasts from breaking down bone. Estrogens, therefore, help conserve bone by reducing bone loss and increasing bone density. The onset of menopause or other causes of decreased estrogen remove this protection.

The advent of menopause accelerates age-related loss of bone mass, with a greater loss in trabecular bone than cortical bone. (You will learn more about the various types of bone in the next chapter.) By contrast, prolonged estrogen exposure, which happens when puberty is early, menopause is late, or a woman uses birth control pills or has had a baby, helps increase and sustain bone. That doesn't mean women should wait until menopause to start taking care of their bones. We teach our children that there are delayed rewards for depositing money into a bank, studying for a test, or training for a competition. We should also teach that their health will profit if they practice life-long behaviors that will decrease their risk for osteoporosis in the future. This includes teaching children how to achieve peak bone mass with regular exercise and a nutritious diet that includes lots of calcium-rich foods.

The percentages of women in the United States who experience natural menopause, by age:

AGE	PERCENTAGE
38	10
44	30
49	50
54	90
58	100

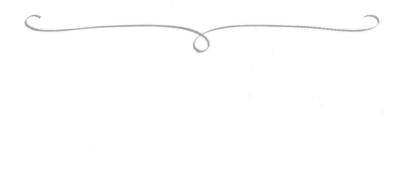

WHAT YOU NEED TO KNOW

Menopause is not the end of a woman's life; it is the beginning of a new phase of her life. Knowledge of what to expect can empower a woman to make the most of it. We are now in an era of health care when physicians' instructions are not blindly accepted. Patients ask questions. Women today do have a say in their physical and emotional well-being. See Appendix E for suggested questions to ask your doctor.

Gaining and Losing Bone

Two-year-old Isabella, one of our younger friends, was in a traumatic accident last year. She was standing near some boards propped against a garage wall, watching her brothers play Ping-Pong. The ball bounced away from the boys and rolled behind the boards. During their enthusiastic pursuit to retrieve the ball, the boys accidentally knocked the boards over on Isabella. She sustained a spiral fracture of her thigh. After surgery to reset the fractured bone, both of Isabella's legs were molded into a plaster cast, rendering her immobile from the waist down for six weeks. It was sad to see this formerly active child lying on her back in a red wagon, pulled by her mother or father from room to room, or lying immobile on the floor, watching videos.

Two weeks later, Isabella was pulling herself everywhere she wanted to go by using the sheer brute force of her arms. She was no longer on painkilling medications, so she slept and woke at normal hours. Although it was a difficult time for Isabella and her family, they were coping.

Only three months after the accident, we were stunned when we visited the family again. Isabella was running all over the place. There were no ill effects from her injury. When asked how Isabella was doing, her mother shrugged her shoulders, shook her head, and replied with amazement, "Great!"

Several years ago Ronda, at age fifty-eight, had a wicked, ankle-twisting fall. She was certain the ankle was broken. It wasn't. Her doctor said that Ronda's active lifestyle had created strong bones that could withstand the violent twisting motion, so that she suffered only a severe sprain. Despite a commitment to her rehabilitation and what her doctor called "a remarkably quick recovery," it was many months before the injury was only a vague memory.

These two incidents are a vivid comparison of how our bodies respond to injury at different ages. We exist in an incredibly efficient machine that constantly builds, breaks down, and repairs tissue throughout life. Unfortunately, as we age, the speed of that process slows down considerably.

Our bones are no exception to this process of change. When we are young and growing, new bone is forming all the time. In adolescence, when children experience accelerated growth spurts, we often hear them complain that their bones ache. This is a sign that the bones are working overtime to lay down new tissue; however, while bone is forming, it is also breaking down. Until we reach our mid-twenties or early thirties, the bone-building exceeds the breakdown process. In our early thirties, bone buildup and breakdown are about equal. Soon breakdown exceeds formation and we begin to lose bone. This constant building and breaking down occurs from the smallest bone in our ear to the largest bone in our thigh.

Even the biggest bones are not hard through and through, because there are two parts to bone. The biggest, which makes up about 80 percent of our skeletal system, is the hard outer bone that protects and supports internal organs and resists the stresses of everyday life. This compact outer bone is called cortical bone. It is what you see when you look at a skeleton. About 80 percent of cortical bone is calcified, which gives it a dense quality.

There is also an inner part of bone called trabecular bone. Only about 20 percent of trabecular bone is calcified. It is more spongy, porous, and flexible than cortical bone. These qualities, like those of a sponge, give it more surface area. Trabecular bone provides the "give" that prevents hard bone from breaking until it is subjected to strong compression or extreme mechanical stress.

There Are Two Parts to Bone:

Cortical bone is the strong, compact outer bone. Bones in the arms, legs, and skull are mostly cortical bone.

Trabecular bone is the spongy, porous, more flexible bone. The ribs, jaw, and spine are mostly trabecular bone.

The lower part of the wrist is about two-thirds trabecular and one-third cortical bone.

When we are infants, none of our bones are hard. They are composed of a rubbery substance called cartilage that, with the exception of the lengthening ends (called epiphyseal growth plates), harden by a process called ossification.

Ossification takes place because bones contain busy cells called osteoblasts. These cells are like masons putting bricks together to build a house. They build (or rebuild) bones that store the calcium and phosphorus (from our diet) that make bones hard. Unless the osteoblasts are diseased, nothing stops these cells from the constant bone-building process.

Osteoblast cells build bones in the same way that masons build walls with mortar and bricks. The calcium- and phosphorus-filled blocks that form bone resemble bricks, and the collagen that cells use to fill the holes resembles mortar. In the same way that more bricks and mortar make a stronger wall, more bone and collagen make stronger bones.

Osteoblasts are stimulated by the female hormone estrogen, the male hormone testosterone, and the growth hormone from the pituitary gland. All act as messengers to tell the osteoblasts to work hard. These hardworking hormones have another supportive tool: calcium. When your body gets enough calcium, the osteoblasts continue to work hard, which encourages an ongoing bone-building cycle.

Like a house that is constantly being remodeled, there is also a demolition and recovery team in the bones. It is composed of other hardworking cells called osteoclasts. Osteoclasts release acids and enzymes, which chew strong bones apart. They deposit the calcium, phosphorus, and protein bone by-products into the bloodstream for use in other parts of the body in a process called resorption. As osteoclasts work, they leave tiny channels behind to be rebuilt by the osteoblasts.

If the osteoblasts work overtime, bones become deformed. If the osteoclasts work overtime, bones become weak.

Remember:

OSTEOBLASTS are BONE BUILDERS
OSTEOCLASTS are BONE BREAKERS

Since the ends of bones are soft, they increase in length until adolescence ends. As we move from adolescence into our mid-twenties, the work of the osteoblasts exceeds that of the osteoclasts. Bones increase in mass, or density, as these bone-building cells build thicker walls. This bone-building process reaches its peak in the trabecular inner bone during our mid-twenties. Our outer cortical bone continues to build, peaking several years later. These early years are the critical times when we have an opportunity to adopt habits that optimize bone health. After this, there is a period of time when bone formation and resorption are about equal.

By our late thirties or early forties, when male and female hormone levels start to decline (long before menopause), resorption starts to accelerate and there is a loss of bone, mostly in the long bones of the arms and legs. The speed of loss is based on genetics and lifestyle factors, including exercise, smoking, diet, and medication. Once a woman begins menopause, her decreased ovarian function reduces the production of estrogen and her bone loss accelerates considerably—about six times more rapidly than a man of the same age. If she does nothing to prevent this loss, her bone—especially the porous trabecular bone—can recede in density to the low levels of childhood.

The Role of Calcium

Throughout life, your body, which considers calcium a pivotal mineral in countless everyday functions, constantly monitors its calcium supply. If you don't have enough calcium in your system because you avoid calcium-rich dairy products, lead a sedentary lifestyle, smoke, drink lots of alcohol, or take corticosteroids or other bone-robbing drugs, your bones get a message that the systems requiring calcium to function optimally must make some adjustments. A kind of telephone tag begins. Low calcium levels trigger the parathyroid gland to secrete a hormone that signals the bone-building osteoblasts to quit storing calcium. The osteoblasts, in turn, tell the osteoclasts to break down bone to release more calcium into the bloodstream. Low calcium levels also signal the kidneys to hold on to any calcium about to be eliminated in urine. Additionally, the kidneys, which have been storing the vitamin D you acquire through sunlight, supplements, or fortified milk, convert those vitamin D stores into an active form called calcitrol. Calcitrol makes the body more efficient at absorbing calcium, making it easier for the parathyroid to get a hormone-based message to the bone.

In addition to its contribution to making the strong bones that form our skeletal system, calcium plays a role in the cardiovascular, muscular, and nervous systems. When women don't get enough calcium in their diet for heart, muscle, and nerve work, the necessary calcium is stolen from the bones.

Calcium
- Keeps nerve impulses flowing
- Allows muscles to contract properly
- Is integral to blood clotting
- Helps regulate hormone balance
- Initiates metabolic pathways

WHAT YOU NEED TO KNOW

If you could look at live bone, you wouldn't see any activity. You might think that it is stable and not very active. Nothing could be further from the truth. Bone is dynamic and alive, actively attempting to maintain the delicate balance between osteoblasts and osteoclasts. The bone-building process, which takes place in both the hard cortical and soft trabecular bone, is at its peak early in life. It is this bone mass attained early in life that may be the most important determinant of life-long skeletal health. A balanced, calcium-rich diet and regular exercise contribute significantly to the efficiency of this process, which peaks at about age thirty. Dietary calcium also plays a role in many physiological functions of the body. When you don't get enough calcium in your diet, the body "steals" calcium from your bones to maintain proper blood calcium levels for "more important" work.

Osteoporosis is not always the result of osteoclast activity. Your early (and current) eating and exercise behaviors, combined with genetics, hormone changes, and other lifestyle factors, determine whether peak bone mass will be maintained. If bone mass is optimized when bone is forming and maintained with healthy lifestyle habits, you will not get osteoporosis unless uncontrollable factors intervene. If bone mass declines until the cortical bone is thin and the once uniform, honeycomb-shaped trabecular bone becomes irregular and enlarged, you will be left with frail bone that is easily fractured; you will be diagnosed with osteoporosis. It's a life-and-death choice you can control. Read on to learn why and how.

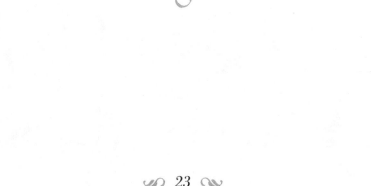

Section II

Your Risk Factors

Uncontrollable Risk Factors

Perhaps your mother or grandmother is like Ruth, whom you met at the beginning of this book. If so, you may be looking into your own future. As you gaze into your crystal ball, do you see brittle bones or a dowager's hump? Do you see yourself afraid to go out because you may fall and break your hip? Before you wrap yourself in foam, let's take a realistic look at your unalterable osteoporosis risk factors.

Why Do Some Women Develop Osteoporosis but Others Do Not?

Many of the reasons why we get osteoporosis can be traced to our ancestors. When it comes to genes, the best thing you can have going for you is an osteoporosis-free family history. We also know that other uncontrollable genetics-related factors, including gender, race, small body frame, or a predisposition to poor calcium absorption, can increase your risk for the disease.

Factors That Encourage Bone Density:
- Parents with strong bones
- Physical activity at every age
- A nutritionally adequate, calcium-rich diet

Factors That Can Foster Bone Loss:

- Menopause
- Age-related bone changes
- Decline in physical activity or no physical activity at a young age
- Impaired absorption of calcium
- Adverse effects of other medical conditions
- Adverse effects of drugs

Risk Factors Explored

Gender

As you learned in chapter 2, being a woman puts you at greater risk for developing osteoporosis. To begin with, women have less bone than men. Women have smaller muscles to move those bones, and they lose bone mass more rapidly than men. There are lots of terrific advantages to being a woman, but your risk for osteoporosis is not one of them.

Race/Ethnicity

Caucasian and Asian women are the most prone to osteoporosis. Studies reveal that fewer African-American, Native-American, and Hispanic women experience the disease; however. they are not without risk and should take the same preventative measures as their more predisposed sisters.

Genetics

Studies of twins and comparisons of mothers and daughters indicate that approximately 60 to 80 percent of the factors contributing to bone density

are genetically determined. If your mother had an osteoporosis-related fracture, your risk for fracture is doubled.

Look at your older relatives for signs that you are vulnerable to this disease. Red flags include any loss of height with aging, curvature of the spine
(dowager's hump), fractures in later years, and/or chronic back pain. (In
chapter 1, you learned that back pain may be one of the first symptoms of
osteoporosis.)

Genetics plays a strong role in the development of many diseases.
Osteoporosis is no exception.

> The siblings of people with osteoporosis are six times more likely
> than the general population to suffer from low bone mineral density.

Bone structure and body weight

Thin, petite women, described by physiologists as ectomorphs, are more
vulnerable to osteoporosis than mesomorphic, bulkier body types. Taller
and heavier women have bigger and denser bones and a lower risk for osteoporosis. Heavier women naturally produce more estrogen from their fat
cells. That gives them more protection against osteoporosis than thin
women, but this advantage over their thinner sisters is slight.

Women with eating disorders, especially anorexia, often have a fragile
body structure and low body weight, both of which give them an appearance
that can be misinterpreted as a genetic predisposition to be small. Scientists
are studying the brain chemistry and certain brain centers of women with
this aberrant lifestyle to determine if there is a genetic and/or biochemical
link that predisposes women to eating disorders. Regardless of the outcome,

eating disorders, crash dieting, overexercising, and a too-lean frame are risk factors for osteoporosis.

> NOTE: Calorie restriction combined with the estrogen deficiency that makes women stop menstruating is a serious threat to current and long-term health.

Medical Issues

Since bones are active, many of the drugs used to systemically treat disease can affect the bones adversely. Additionally, diseases that don't appear to affect bones may be silently doing damage.

> A recent review by the National Institute of Mental Health (NIMH) of published research underscored the serious ramifications of depression, when it revealed that women who had experienced a lengthy bout of depression also had low bone density. It is believed that the higher levels of the hormone cortisol associated with depression decreases osteoblastic activity. The report indicated that as many as 400,000 depressed women in their thirties and forties may also have brittle bones.

What Is a Woman to Do?

If you are like us, daughters of women with osteoporosis, you may wonder, "Am I doomed to get osteoporosis?"

The answer is no. You have the power to overcome a genetic, racial, or gender-based predisposition for osteoporosis by addressing the risk factors you *can* control. While you practice healthy, osteoporosis-preventing behaviors, scientists are hard at work searching for drugs to cure this disease. Scientists are attempting to identify a specific gene for osteoporosis. It would be wonderful if we could be tested at an early age to discover if we are at risk for osteoporosis—much as women whose mothers died of breast cancer can be tested today. Women who are adopted or whose mothers died at an early age could gain information not currently available to them. So far, the resulting data for an osteoporosis gene are unclear. In the meantime, read on to learn about other risk factors, testing, and treatment for osteoporosis, and the prevention strategies that will make you a smart woman with strong bones and help you outwit osteoporosis.

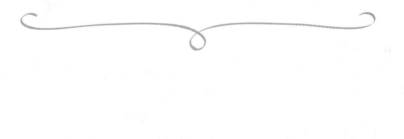

WHAT YOU NEED TO KNOW

Although it's impossible to change your gender, race, frame size, or family history of osteoporosis, you are not doomed to repeat the past. There are alterable risk factors for osteoporosis that can change your predisposition to this disease. If you make them a priority now, your future can be a healthy one.

Controllable Risk Factors

Psychologists have gone to great lengths to attempt to understand why people engage in behaviors that are not in their best interests. We have learned that these self-defeating behaviors are usually initiated when we are under stress or when we feel vulnerable. When we exercise these behaviors, we feel better for a short period of time (the payoff) but later feel guilty about doing something that wasn't in our best interests (the price). In time, because these behaviors can be controlled, many of us are able to overcome them. This liberation from self-defeating behaviors changes our lives. Sadly, before we are able to control or manage these behaviors, they can compromise our physical health. This can include ongoing detrimental physical changes we cannot see because they occur deep inside our bodies. Some of these behaviors affect our bones. Consider your own lifestyle as you review some of these controllable risk factors.

Diet

If you could see a human metabolism chart, you might be surprised to learn how essential vitamins and minerals are to life. They play a vital role in every cell. They help move oxygen through your blood, build cells for your eyes, help muscles contract, and increase the density of your bones.

Suddenly it becomes easier to understand why it is important for children to have an adequate diet. When children are deprived of the vitamins and minerals they need to grow, they have a delayed puberty. That creates risk factors for many diseases later in life, including osteoporosis. Although all nutrients are important, the need for calcium to provide early prevention against osteoporosis is sufficient reason for us to tell children, "Drink your milk."

There are many resources that explore in depth the connection between diet and osteoporosis. In the United States, the American Dairy Council and its state organizations do a terrific job of teaching kids of all ages about the benefits of dairy products. You can also consult your library or the Internet for additional resources.

As we move through puberty to adulthood, up to 2 percent of our total body weight is the calcium in our bones. That calcium comes from our diet. This is why it is important for adults, as well as for children, to consume dairy products. Despite this knowledge, many "experts" tell us we don't need to drink milk after puberty. We hear, "Animals don't drink milk after they are weaned, so why should humans?" That argument is insane. Think about it. Female animals don't have to worry about menopause. They are physically active. They don't live long enough to get osteoporosis. *Women do!*

If you don't drink milk, you need to be more aggressive about getting your calcium from other dairy products and other calcium-rich or calcium-fortified foods. If you choose a milk-free diet because you are lactose intolerant, there are over-the-counter products at your drugstore that can relieve the gas caused by your body's inability to break down milk sugars. Bottom line: If dairy products aren't a part of your diet, it is essential that you work with a dietitian to be sure you get the nutrients you are missing when you eliminate this food group from your diet. If you don't, you could pay with your life.

High-Protein Diets

As this book goes to press, there is a resurgence in the promotion of high-protein diets for weight loss. Although there are hundreds of studies that prove weight management is about balancing calories in and calories out, we continue to hear from hucksters who have their pocketbooks, not your health, as their motivation for perpetuating crash diet myths.

Most Americans already eat much more protein than their bodies need. When they do, their bodies must metabolize the excess. Proteins are nothing more than a group of amino acids. Osteoclasts remove bone more easily in an acid environment. You can see how a high-protein diet that puts lots of amino acids into the blood could set the bone-depleting osteoclastic activity, described in chapter 3, in motion. This cycle can be a setup for an increased risk of osteoporosis, especially if it is combined with a low intake of calcium-rich foods.

> Women who buy into the high-protein diet weight-loss strategy should be aware that it can be dangerous to their bones.

Interestingly, some studies show that vegetarians have a lower incidence of osteoporosis than meat eaters. Although the jury is still out and other factors could be involved (do vegetarians, as a group, exercise more or smoke less than meat eaters?), this relationship is of interest to those of us eager to learn everything we can about preventing this tragic disease.

Eating Disorders

If you have ever stood in line to pay for groceries, you know that the covers of most popular women's magazines are graced by excessively thin models or media personalities. These magazines feature articles that promise to reveal the secret to permanent weight loss, how to dress to camouflage figure flaws, or how to cook meals that reflect the latest diet craze. Many of us tell others we think these media-driven messages to be thin are a travesty, but we also find ourselves worrying about our weight and beating ourselves up for enjoying a high-calorie dessert. Women who take the "thin is better" message too far and develop an eating disorder seriously compromise their mental, emotional, and physical well-being—including their gynecological and bone health.

Bulimia

Bulimia is a "binge and purge" eating disorder. It is characterized by eating excessive amounts of food in a short period of time. Gorging typically continues until it is interrupted by the severe discomfort of feeling full. This awareness triggers an intense fear of weight gain that precipitates self-induced vomiting, fasting, abuse of laxatives, use of diet pills or diuretics, and excessive exercise.

Bulimia is a serious health problem that most frequently affects women in late adolescence or young adulthood. Its cause is complex, and since people with bulimia are usually of normal weight, it often goes unrecognized.

When a woman continues a cycle of bingeing and purging, her body becomes depleted of water, potassium, and other minerals, including bone-building calcium. As this disease progresses, the body responds by making adjustments in all systems, including the reproductive system. Estrogen levels decrease and menstruation becomes irregular or ceases. This contributes further to the failure to build strong bones. Osteoporosis is almost a certainty.

Exercise bulimia

Exercise bulimia is a lesser-known form of bulimia that is characterized by a food intake–exercise relationship designed to maintain weight. People who suffer from exercise bulimia are terrified of getting fat. The potential enjoyment of each meal is tempered by obsessive thoughts and accompanied by a plan for the exercise that must follow to prevent any fat storage. People who suffer from exercise bulimia have an appearance of good health and physical fitness, but their exercise has nothing to do with health benefits. Sadly, the fitness community often supports this disease. Exercise instructors often encourage their clients to exercise to "burn off those calories" eaten at an earlier meal or to create the calorie deficit that gives them permission to eat more at the next meal. Most active women who have issues about their body image or weight practice some form of exercise bulimia, which has erroneously been described as a positive addiction. This is an oxymoron. Although exercise bulimia doesn't directly precipitate osteoporosis, it is often one of the steps that leads to the bone-robbing diseases of bulimia and anorexia. It is also an acceptable "recovery" route for former bulimics.

Anorexia nervosa

Anorexia nervosa is a more serious eating disorder believed to be rooted in issues of control. When a woman feels out of control, one of the things she *can* control is what she eats. If that woman also has an unrealistic self-perception of body size and a fear of being fat, she is at risk for the self-starvation syndrome known as anorexia. These women have a pre-occupation with calorie counting and food preparation. They are often great cooks who encourage others to eat but rarely swallow anything themselves. If you watch them during a meal, you will see they are just pushing food around on their plate. Their severe restriction of food intake leads to dramatic weight loss. Soon there is a loss of muscle, which gives them an emaciated look. Anorexia is most common in adolescent girls and young women whose physically small appearance may also represent an attempt to avoid the responsibility of adulthood. It is also a well-known occupational hazard for people in the media, where cameras can make them look heavier than they are, and in the dance community, where many choreographers want their dancers to be skinny and birdlike. These women on pointed toe often experience fractures of their fragile feet and legs.

An irregular or nonexistent menstrual cycle is one of the diagnostic criteria for anorexia. The risk for fracture later in life for women with anorexia is twice that of their healthy peers. Anorexia is one of the most difficult eating disorders to treat. A woman who recovers and adopts a proper diet will regain weight, but she will have no improvement in bone mass—even if she takes bone-building estrogen.

Despite recent books and articles explaining that women who struggle with eating disorders pay a heavy psychological and physiological price for their behavior, it's difficult for them to grasp the concept that this price may not be visible for many years. As women age, they are challenged by the body changes that occur with decreased physical activity, especially when it coincides with menopause. This challenge, coupled with the belief that women cannot be too thin, drives too many of us toward dangerous consequences, including fragile bones.

> Excessive pursuit of thinness permanently affects bone health.

Exercise

Ask anyone you meet, "Is exercise important to good health?" Unless they've been in a cave, their answer will be yes, even if they don't exercise. Study after study reaffirms the benefits of exercise. In unearthing ancient skeletons, anthropologists have discovered that one forearm bone of those skeletons was enlarged, which led them to conclude that slinging spears, boomerangs, bolas, and stones exercised the muscles and strengthened the bones in the dominant arm. Pay attention! People who exercise have denser and stronger bones. And positive changes take place in all people who exercise, regardless of the age at which they start exercising regularly.

If lack of exercise is such a significant predictor for developing osteoporosis, why do so many women procrastinate?

> An active lifestyle in the early years of life encourages bone density.
> An active lifestyle in the middle and later years of life retains or rebuilds bone density.

Perhaps too many of us remember exercise experiences based on the mantra of early fitness gurus who preached the "No pain, no gain" message. It may have been the operating guideline when the exercise instructor stereotype was a drill sergeant with a clipboard and whistle, but it is no longer true. Bone-building exercise requires effort, but it shouldn't be painful. Today's mantra is "Use it or lose it."

Everyone has a busy life filled with commitments. "I don't have time" is the typical excuse. Consider this: If you wanted to lose a dress size for your high school reunion, wouldn't you make time to exercise? If you knew a big deposit in your bank account would be the reward for an investment in exercise, wouldn't you adjust your priorities?

We remind people, "If you don't exercise now, you may not be able to participate in the activities you can enjoy later in life." Too often we hear, "That's OK. I deserve to sit around later." Then later comes, and with it the pain of fragile bones and a dowager's hump, both of which make sitting around painful.

There is one population group that does not benefit from exercise. Women who exercise so much that they stop menstruating (a condition called amenorrhea) have very low levels of estrogen. It is as though the body says, "You can't exercise so much and maintain the resources to support a new life." Studies show that these women have a significantly lower mineral density in the spine along the lower back. If these women stop overexercising and are treated with hormone replacement therapy, they will maintain the bone they have, but they will not replace the lost bone.

Doctors agree that if exercise could be packaged in a pill, it would be the most prescribed drug in the world today. Take our advice: Climb steps, lift weights, use a treadmill, or take a long walk in the fresh air. Your bones will love it.

Caffeine

If caffeine were discovered today, it would be banned from our diet because of its extraordinary addictive properties. It sends us racing to the bathroom; it keeps us awake. Nevertheless, we are willing to spend several dollars a day to get our physical and physiological fix. No substance has been the subject of more urgent health bulletins—all mutually contradictory—than caffeine.

Researchers continue to attempt to clarify conflicting research about links between caffeine and cancer, caffeine and heart disease, and caffeine and osteoporosis. One study calculated that calcium loss from the use of as little as 40 mg of caffeine a day added up to a 10 to 15 percent bone loss per decade. Another study refuted the first when the subjects chosen didn't smoke or use alcohol; however, since people who exercise rarely smoke and often choose to avoid alcohol, these factors could have accounted for the difference in the studies.

If you prefer caffeinated coffee or tea, consider adding extra milk to offset the calcium-draining effects of caffeine.

Only 300 mg of caffeine (about two cups of coffee) can cause your body to excrete 15 mg of calcium and other important minerals. This amount may seem insignificant when we consider that total calcium makes up about 2 percent of our body weight. But since little things can add up, it is wise for people at risk for osteoporosis, especially older women, to go the non-caffeine route as often as possible.

Caffeine: Is It Worth the Lift?

Source	*Milligrams of caffeine*
Cola (12 oz.)	
Jolt Cola®	100
Sugar-free Mr. Pibb®	58.8
Mountain Dew®	54
Tab®	46.8
Coca-Cola®	45.6
Diet Coke®	45.6
Pepsi®	38.4
Coffee and Tea	
6 oz. fresh drip coffee	115–175
6 oz. brewed coffee	90–140
6 oz. instant coffee	66–100
6 oz. decaffeinated coffee	2–4
6 oz. hot tea	30–100
1.5 oz. espresso	100
12 oz. iced tea	70
Chocolate	
1 oz. chocolate bar	15
1 oz. baking chocolate, unsweetened	25
Painkillers (per pill)	
Excedrin®	65
Anacin®	32
Cold medications	varies; see label
Other Over-the-Counter Pills (per pill)	
Vivarin®	100
NoDoz®	100

Smoking

Back when it was cool to smoke, we saw older, dowager-humped women sitting around with cigarettes hanging out of their mouths. They knew about the addictive properties of nicotine but had little awareness that their habit was precipitating wrinkles and fragile bones.

Cigarettes deactivate your production of estrogen. (Remember, estrogen encourages osteoblasts to build bones.) Women who smoke tend to go through menopause earlier than women who don't smoke, adding extra years of low estrogen production and, subsequently, more bone loss.

If you used to smoke and are now smoke-free, good for you. If you haven't given up nicotine yet, try one of the excellent smoke cessation programs available. End your use of this life-threatening drug. The resource section in the appendix of this book has a few suggestions.

Alcohol

If you enjoy a glass or two of wine with dinner, you probably cheered when research revealed that a moderate consumption of alcohol can have a positive effect on heart health. This news is a good example of one of our favorite sayings, "Statistics are like bikinis; they reveal only part of the truth." What the highly publicized media reports forgot to add is that a little alcohol may support good health, but a lot of alcohol interferes with calcium absorption, increasing the risk of osteoporosis. A review of the health charts of alcoholics reveals the truth: Alcoholics have a much higher incidence of osteoporosis than nondrinkers. Alcoholics tend to drink their calories and have a diet that is low in vitamins and minerals. The figure of speech "falling-down drunk" can have severe repercussions for women whose bones get fragile because they overuse, abuse, or become addicted to this potent drug. Enjoy an occasional glass or two of wine or beer, but remember, moderation in all things is the best course of action.

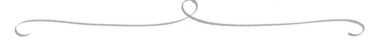

WHAT YOU NEED TO KNOW

Most people who want to change self-defeating behaviors (including yo-yo dieting, failing to exercise, too much coffee, smoking, or alcohol) say, "I know what I need to do, but I just can't seem to do it." The compulsive quality of all these behaviors has repercussions in all areas of life. In short, if you want to be active and bone healthy in your elder years, you must take responsibility for your errant ways today, not tomorrow. Every moment counts.

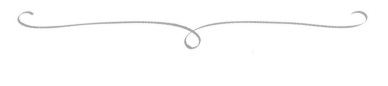

Drugs and Medications

Do You Use Drugs?

Your first reaction to this question may be a resolute "no," because this question often refers to drugs that are self-administered and abused. Popping a variety of pills and potions every day is so common that most of us think nothing of it. Whether in the form of an over-the-counter purchase to alleviate a minor symptom; a prescription from your physician to prevent or treat a disease; or food, herbs, or other supplements, drug use has become a part of modern life.

When taken as directed, prescription and nonprescription drugs, supplements, and foods can effectively treat many symptoms and illnesses. That is the good news. There is accompanying bad news: Most medication works on more than one site or system of the body. For every positive action derived from the use of a drug there is almost always an accompanying message to the brain and body that elicits an unrecognized or unwanted response.

Ruth, whom you met in our preface, took thyroid medication after she received a diagnosis of hypothyroidism (an underactive thyroid) in her mid-thirties. The prescription stabilized her symptoms; however, the blood tests available at that time to determine an appropriate dose could only tell the doctor if she was receiving too little thyroid medication. Recently developed tests to measure thyroid are much more sophisticated. They include a test that measures the amount of thyroid-stimulating hormone (TSH) in the blood. A high TSH means thyroid production is low; dosage is increased. If TSH is low, the patient is getting too much thyroid medication. By the time Ruth's TSH revealed her current dose could be lowered, she had already had more than twenty years of excessive therapy in her system. That unnecessary medication contributed to her fragile bones and set the stage for the compression fractures of her spine at age eighty.

There are many medicines, in addition to thyroid medication, that have undesirable effects on the health of our bones. Because you often need these medicines to treat other diseases, it is important to understand which of the drugs that you use also affect bones, so you can be more diligent about taking the necessary steps to prevent osteoporosis.

Every drug that has a benefit almost always has a liability. Patients must always weigh the pros and cons of treatment with their doctor.

Bone-Busting Drugs
Thyroid Medications
The endocrine glands in our bodies are very tiny, but they pack a powerful punch. The thyroid may be the most powerful of all. This two-lobed gland is about the size of a thumb. It sits on the front of the lower part of the neck. The thyroid gland produces three hormones that are important for the function we call metabolism. The amount of hormone produced by the thyroid is regulated by the thyroid stimulating hormone, which is located in another

powerful gland called the pituitary. If your thyroid is overstimulated, the diagnosis is hyperthyroidism—a syndrome marked by a fast metabolism that can make you feel very energetic, give you a slight hand tremor, and cause you to lose weight. If your thyroid is understimulated, your diagnosis is hypothyroidism—a syndrome that can make you feel very sluggish and cause weight gain.

For a long time, thyroid medication was extracted from the thyroid glands of cows. It was difficult to regulate the dose. Now most doctors use one of the many synthetic thyroid extracts that delivers that missing punch. The correct dose for each patient is precisely regulated based on a blood test that measures levels of TSH. If the TSH is low, the doctor knows that the patient is getting too much thyroid, and he or she can adjust the dose until TSH levels become normal. Then thyroid-induced osteoporosis is no longer a risk.

If you feel tired and sluggish and know you are perimenopausal or menopausal, be sure to report these symptoms to your doctor. Your blood will be drawn and a TSH test ordered to discover whether the cause of your symptoms is hypothyroidism. If it is, you will receive a prescription for medication you should take daily. A follow-up blood test will be scheduled to make sure your thyroid is at optimum function but not compromising the health of your bones.

Corticosteroids

The term corticosteroids (sometimes called adrenocorticosteroids, or simply steroids) describes many powerful drugs that mimic the action of the adrenal glands. These two small glands, about the size of the end section of your thumb, sit on top of your kidneys. They produce cortisone-like chemicals, including sex hormones, hormones that convert starchy foods into glucose (the storage form of sugar), and hormones that maintain fluid balance and reduce inflammation. If you have an adrenal deficiency (Addison's Disease) or a disease, such as lupus or arthritis, the long-term use of corticosteroids will reduce swelling, pain, redness, and heat. Corticosteroids are also used to treat asthma, certain skin diseases, and some cancers.

In the short term (for a week or two), oral use of corticosteroids, injection of the drug into a joint or excessive scar tissue, or use of topical preparations will produce the desired effect of the drug with no residual side effects. However, multiple short treatments or long-term use of these remarkable medications by people who have normal adrenal function can decrease the action of bone-forming osteoblasts and the absorption of calcium, effects that can last for a long time after the drug has been discontinued. The urine of people who use corticosteroids shows an increased amount of calcium, indicating that there is an ongoing increase in bone loss. In other words, corticosteroids destroy the bone-building and enhance the bone-breakdown process. This produces a potentially severe bone loss that makes the spine and ribs susceptible to fractures with the slightest trauma.

If your doctor prescribes cortisone, hydrocortisone, or one of their modified forms, like prednisone (5 mg or more for over two months), you need to be sure you are practicing as many bone-loss prevention strategies as possible. (See chapters 12–15.)

Asthmatic children who use steroid inhalants that ease the constriction in their lungs are at great risk for osteoporosis at an early age.

Never stop taking steroids just because you read that they can harm your bones. Instead, talk with your doctor about the appropriateness of the dose and the expected duration of your treatment.

The more common steroid prescription drugs are:

Aristocort®	Cortisone®	Depo-Provera®	Prednisone
Celestone®	Decadron®	Medrol®	
Cortef®	Deltasone®	Prednisolone	

Steroids for Birth Control

There are research studies that report that the use of the injectable contraceptive Depo-Provera® (medroxyprogesterone acetate, or DMPA), which depresses estrogen production, is associated with significant loss of bone density, most of which is reversible after the drug is discontinued.

Diuretics

Diuretics are drugs that increase urine volume. They are prescribed to treat high blood pressure and congestive heart failure by decreasing blood volume and, subsequently, the workload of the heart. Like most drugs, there are several classes of diuretics. Only one class, the loop diuretics (which get their name because they work in an area of the kidney called Henle's Loop), cause the kidney to excrete excess calcium. Loop diuretics are so good at removing calcium from the body that they are prescribed for people whose calcium levels get too high. If you take Lasix,® Aldactone,® Dyazide,® Bumes,® Diamox,® or Edecrin,® you need to drink additional water, add extra calcium to your diet, and, with your doctor's permission, participate in an ongoing exercise program.

Anticonvulsants

The brain is a remarkable organ. It transmits millions of electric-like charges and signals that regulate conscious and unconscious thoughts, feelings, and actions. When these signals become disorganized, the result is a seizure or convulsion. Epilepsy is the most commonly known long-term seizure disorder.

Anticonvulsant medication prevents seizures by inhibiting the repetitive spread of electrical impulses along nerve pathways. It also affects the liver's metabolism of vitamin D. When vitamin D isn't metabolized properly, the body doesn't absorb calcium very well.

The most commonly-used anticonvulsant is phenytoin (trade name Dilantin®). Phenobarbital, which is used less often, has the same effect. Since these drugs are taken for a lifetime, their use is a risk factor for osteoporosis. Patients who use them should take a calcium and vitamin D supplement.

Antacids

If you suffer from acid indigestion, gastric reflux disease, or ulcers, you may be using an antacid to neutralize the excess gastric secretions that irritate tissues and cause abdominal pain. Some of these antacids are salts derived from mineral sources, including aluminum. When you take an aluminum-based antacid, your body isn't able to absorb the bone-building calcium and phosphate from your diet. Occasional use of aluminum-based antacids is not a risk factor for osteoporosis; however, if you use them every day, you may get relief from pain but your bones will pay the consequences. Non–aluminum-based antacids do not have this bone-depleting effect.

Aluminum-based Antacids	Non–aluminum-based Antacids
Aludros®	Alka-Seltzer®
Amphojel®	Bisodol®
Gaviscon®	Mylicon®
Gelusil®	Rolaids®*
Kolantyl®	Titralac®*
Maalox®	Tums®*
Mylanta®	
Riopan®	

NOTE: This list is not intended to be a complete list of all aluminum-containing antacids. Check with your pharmacist or look at the label on the product you use.

*These antacids contain calcium carbonate. Their supplemental use is beneficial to bones.

Other Drugs Used Less Often
Lithium

One of the great advances in modern society is the acceptance that mental illnesses, which once sent us to institutions or ostracized us from society, are often biochemically based. Many mental illnesses can now be tempered with a combination of drugs and behavior therapy. One of these miracle drugs is Lithium. Lithium is used to treat bipolar disorder, a syndrome marked by wide mood swings.

Lithium tempers these profound mental disturbances, but, like many drugs, it has side effects. In this case it is increased production of parathyroid hormone, which plays a role in the breakdown of bone. If Lithium has been prescribed for you, it is important that your mental health program includes a physical activity program to keep your bones strong.

Heparin

Heparin is a blood thinner used to prevent or treat life-threatening blood clots. It is rarely administered outside of a hospital setting. People who need to take this injection daily for an extended period of time have an increased risk of osteoporosis. Once again, the benefits of the drug far outweigh the risks, but if you need to use heparin for a long time, talk to your doctor about bone protection strategies.

Drugs that treat breast cancer

Ronda's friend Nancy, a five-foot-tall bundle of energy on a small frame, was recently diagnosed with breast cancer. Nancy's short stature and small build put her at risk for osteoporosis. Her active lifestyle, which included teaching fitness classes, cycling, hiking, and skiing, kept her bones strong—until she was treated for breast cancer.

When her course of treatment was over, Nancy celebrated a full return to her pre-diagnosis lifestyle. Her doctor did not mention a post-treatment risk for osteoporosis, so she didn't think twice about the possibility that she might experience a fracture. One day while skiing she took a fall that would not break an average person's bones, but it broke Nancy's leg in several places. Her recovery included months in a wheelchair, physical therapy, and a slow resumption of her physical strength. Happily, Nancy has fully recovered. Like most breast cancer survivors, she is not a candidate for estrogen therapy to treat her osteoporosis, so she is on one of the drugs you will learn about in chapter 9. Her warning to all women with breast cancer, "Be sure to have a bone scan before and after chemotherapy," is now supported by most oncologists.

Drugs that treat any cancer prolong and save lives. Like many drugs that produce strong therapeutic responses to temper or cure a disease, they may have long-term side effects. When a premenopausal woman receives chemotherapy for breast cancer, there can be a premature and abrupt shutdown of estrogen production, which can rapidly deplete up to 8 percent of bone mass. Women over forty, whose ovaries are already producing less estrogen, are more vulnerable to this side effect of chemotherapy. Nancy's multiple fracture experience was undoubtedly a result of a similar bone loss.

Dr. Marisa Weiss, founder of www.breastcancer.org, tells us that not all drug combinations used to treat breast cancer precipitate menopause, although it is quite common for menstruation to become irregular or stop during the course of treatment. Early menopause is more likely with a combination of cyclophosphamide, methotrexate, and fluorouracil (CMF) than it is with one of the many regimens that contain Adriamycin® (doxorubicin). Tamoxifen,® a drug used after chemotherapy to prevent recurrence of cancer, helps protect bone but can also produce the symptoms of menopause.

It is not unusual for someone who is treated with these powerful medications to become vulnerable to fractures. Since the drugs are crucial for survival and their benefits far outweigh their many side effects, there is little interest in researching how these drugs harm bones.

Dr. Weiss reminds us that sound nutrition and exercise, in keeping with physical stamina, are critical to the treatment for cancer (or for any disease).

She prescribes a calcium and vitamin D regimen as part of the treatment for her breast cancer patients. At www.breastcancer.org, a patient will receive advice on how to make important lifestyle changes during the course of her cancer treatment that concurs with the advice in this book. Patients are encouraged to get a pretherapy baseline bone density study, followed by a repeat assessment if their menstrual cycle stops for more than three months or doesn't resume after treatment. If the results show a loss of bone strength, one of the many non–estrogen-related drugs that help build bone and keep it strong (see chapter 9) may be prescribed. Most important for breast cancer survivors is the need for open dialogue with their doctors and equal partnership with them in their treatment.

WHAT YOU NEED TO KNOW

There are a variety of illnesses that call for a prescription or an over-the-counter medication that can weaken bones or aggravate existing or undiagnosed osteoporosis. As you age, you are likely to use more pills and potions on a regular basis, so you must be cognizant of the undesirable effects of these treatments. If you take any medicine for a long period of time, be sure to ask your physician or pharmacist if the drugs that are helping you might also be harming your bones.

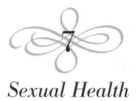

Sexual Health

Can your sexual health really affect your bones? Once you understand that sexual (reproductive) organs and sexual events (e.g., the age at which menstrual periods begin) depend on estrogen (and progesterone and testosterone), the answer obviously becomes "Yes, it can."

Periods Stopped for an Extended Time

There are a number of reasons why a woman's menstrual cycle can become irregular or stop completely (amenorrhea). When this happens, there are tremendous fluctuations in sexual hormones that can affect bones. In pregnancy this is a good change for bones. The hormones combined with the nutrients from food the mother eats build bones for her baby and for herself. The weight she gains puts additional pressure on her bones, which increases their density. Other disturbances in the menstrual cycle are not so beneficial for women. They create a risk for osteopenia and for osteoporosis itself.

Women who are amenorrheic at any time (except pregnancy) are vulnerable to osteoporosis.

Anorexia Nervosa and Bulimia

Although these eating disorders (described in chapter 5) are seen in women more often than in men, we don't know if they are related to the sex hormones. Nevertheless, one of the diagnostic criteria for anorexia is cessation of menses. Most long-term bulimics and anorexics do not have normal menstrual cycles. If you don't eat or if you binge and purge, your bones will suffer the consequences.

Female Athletes

Many competitive female athletes are amenorrheic. Think about it: If a woman is training really hard, it is stressful to her body. The body says, "Your effort to reach a high level of fitness overrides my need to support new life." Estrogen levels decline. You would think that their high level of physical training would overcome this low estrogen effect on their bones. It doesn't.

If these women are treated with hormone replacement therapy, they maintain current bone mineral density but bone replacement does not occur. Nevertheless, we have yet to meet a highly competitive athlete who makes osteoporosis prevention a higher priority than winning a race. These women train hard. They take their vitamins. They eat a healthy diet to improve performance. Because their "work out to compete" lifestyle contributes to low estrogen levels, they put themselves at risk for developing fractures later in life.

Other Bone Makers and Bone Breakers
Disturbances in Ovulation

Women who have ovulatory disturbances without amenorrhea, meaning that they have menstrual periods but do not ovulate, also have deficits in bone mass. This bone loss, which may be due to inadequate production of progesterone, is estimated to be 4.2 percent a year.

No Children

Women who have not given birth to children, by choice or because of fertility problems, seem to be at greater risk for osteoporosis. The reasons for this are not clear. It's possible they simply don't experience the bone-building hormonal surges shared by women who experience pregnancy.

Onset of Menstruation

Women who have an early onset of puberty and begin menstruating early have greater bone mass than women who begin menstruating in their late teens. Scientists believe it is because they have more estrogen circulating in their body for a longer period of time.

Hysterectomy

Pre-menopausal women who have had a hysterectomy without the removal of their ovaries have significantly lower bone density than normally menstruating women. It is not known if this bone loss occurs because the uterus was removed or simply because the ovaries are no longer functioning properly.

Extended Lactation

Although we don't know why mothers who breastfeed have bone loss, studies show it does occur. Typically, bone density improves and returns to pre-pregnancy levels within a year after a woman gives birth. When breastfeeding continues longer than a year, this return of bone density to pre-pregnancy levels does not occur. Hopefully, new safe drug strategies will emerge that can overcome the bone-weakening effects of a mother's desire to breastfeed her baby for a long time.

Early Menopause

As you already know, menopause is characterized by the loss of estrogen production by the ovaries. When the natural onset of menopause comes earlier than expected or when it is induced surgically by removal of the ovaries, a woman's level of bone-supportive estrogen is reduced for a longer period of time. Women whose ovaries are removed surgically can show signs of osteoporosis within two years if they do not receive hormone replacement therapy (HRT). That is why women who have early menopause and do not take HRT are at an increased risk for osteoporosis.

Sexual Exercise

You have learned about the role of alterable risk factors, which include weight-bearing exercise, on bone density. Well, what about sexual exercise? Beverly, who coauthored the best-selling book *The G Spot* and has written more than 125 research articles about sexuality, reminds us that depending on the positions used during sexual intercourse, a woman can participate in weight-bearing or non–weight-bearing exercise with a loved one. Sexual encounters are supposed to be good for you. Be creative. Enjoy it. Think of and use intercourse positions that help provide weight-bearing sexual activity and enjoyment for you and your lover.

Sexual Dysfunction and Your Bones

You may be surprised to learn that more than 40 percent of women report a sexual problem at some time in their lives. Two of the problems are diminished sexual desire and a noticeable lack of lubrication. These two problems may be related to lower levels of estrogen in the body. The decrease in vaginal lubrication may occur because as estrogen declines there is a reduced blood flow to the vagina. The wall of the vaginal lining becomes thinner, and painful intercourse is the result. These changes may begin at the same time as bone mass loss begins (the late thirties or forties). Burning and pain during intercourse can begin long before a gynecologist is able to detect changes in the vagina. If pain during intercourse is a problem for you, use a water-based lubricant and consider HRT. Painful intercourse is not normal at any age. If you experience it, be sure to see your health-care provider.

A decrease in sexual desire can be related to other symptoms of perimenopause. When you are experiencing insomnia, night sweats, hot flashes, and irritability, a sexual lifestyle isn't a high priority. HRT not only helps prevent osteoporosis but it also increases vaginal lubrication and sexual desire. Studies also support the message that women who masturbate or have intercourse regularly (once a week or more) have twice as much circulating estrogen as women who are not sexually active or active only sporadically. There's much to support the axiom "use it or lose it."

In short, you can have a healthy sexual life and prevent osteoporosis at the same time.

WHAT YOU NEED TO KNOW

Some of the sexual lifestyle choices that women make may affect their risk for osteoporosis. Any choice that decreases the amount of estrogen circulating in the body puts a woman at risk for osteoporosis. Not having children, extended breastfeeding, early menopause, or surgical menopause without HRT are a few examples. An active sex life, including weight-bearing sexual activity, is a good prescription for bone health.

Section III

What You Can Do

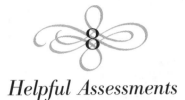

Helpful Assessments

We meet too many women who worry about getting old. They believe aging means a less meaningful, less functional, and less productive life, and that those extra birthday candles will provoke poor health. Many women fear the dowager's hump of osteoporosis. We believe that women need to alter their perspective and look at the assets the aging process and maturity can bring to their lives.

When it comes to osteoporosis, repeat the following: "Deteriorating bones are not inevitable." Today's woman can prevent, and even reverse, bone loss by learning early—before she breaks a bone or shrinks in height—whether she is losing bone. All it takes is a visit to her doctor who, in most cases, will recommend tests to detect her risk for osteoporosis. With this information in hand, she and her health-care provider can make informed decisions regarding treatment of any existing disease and prevention of future bone loss. This is particularly important if she is struggling with a decision regarding the benefits and/or risks of hormone replacement therapy (HRT).

There are several useful and other not-so-useful tests to help in this decision-making process.

Tests that Diagnose Osteoporosis

The best tool to diagnose brittle bones (95 percent accurate) is called a bone mineral density (BMD) test. BMD testing can:

- Establish the diagnosis of osteoporosis
- Confirm the diagnosis in a person with a "fragility fracture"
- Predict any future fracture risk
- Monitor the progression of a diagnosed case of osteoporosis
- Monitor the effects of therapy to halt or reverse osteoporosis

We agree with recommendations of the National Osteoporosis Foundation and other health organizations, which recommend BMD testing for:

- All postmenopausal women under age sixty-five who have at least one risk factor (including use of certain medications such as steroids or thyroid replacement therapy, eating disorders, a family history of osteoporosis, smoking, a small frame, excessive alcohol intake, poor diet, excessive dieting, or lifelong low calcium intake)
- All women over age sixty-five
- Postmenopausal women who have had a bone fracture
- Women on HRT, steroids, or thyroid medication for a prolonged period of time

Any woman who stops taking HRT should talk to her doctor about whether she needs a BMD.

If you have had any fractures, be sure to ask your doctor for a BMD assessment. Although doctors are becoming more savvy about the relationship between fractures and osteoporosis, a recent study of women over age fifty-four who suffered a wrist fracture revealed that only one-third were given a follow-up bone density scan to determine if the fracture was osteoporosis related. If you break a bone, be sure to ask your doctor, "Could this be an indication I'm at risk for osteoporosis?"

There are several methods for measuring BMD.

DEXA Scan

The preferred method for measurement of BMD is dual-energy X ray absorptiometry (DXA or DEXA). DEXA is the most widely used and most accurate procedure for measuring bone density in clinical practice and research. DEXA measures BMD in the spine, hip, or wrist, the most common sites for osteoporotic fractures. A DEXA scan requires no pills or injections. It is painless and can be completed in less than fifteen minutes. The radiation exposure is approximately one-tenth that of a standard chest X ray. You will get more radiation during a plane ride than from a DEXA scan.

If you are scheduled for this assessment, you will be able to eat before you go, but you will be instructed not to take a calcium supplement for twenty-four hours prior to your appointment. Some calcium supplements dissolve more slowly than others (more about that in chapter 13). If yours is a slow-absorbing variety that remains in your intestines when the DEXA is taken, you may get a false result.

When you arrive at the DEXA testing facility, you will be escorted into an imaging room. You will be asked a series of questions that review the risk factors for osteoporosis. Then you will be instructed to lie, fully clothed, on a padded table. (If you have an item of clothing with metal zippers near your hip or waist, you will be asked to remove it.) A technician will position your body accurately; then a computerized scanner will be activated to automatically record the necessary images.

A DEXA scan typically costs $100 to $500 or more, which includes the fee for the radiologist who interprets the scan. Nevertheless, it's the assessment of choice because it is more comprehensive than other less expensive techniques. In 1994 there were 750 DEXA machines in the United States. As this book goes to press, there are more than four thousand machines in facilities nationwide.

> If you have a diagnosis of breast cancer, put a DEXA scan near the top of your "to do" list before and after treatment. You can't afford to lose bone mass, since estrogen replacement therapy is not one of your treatment options.

SXA Scan

Single-energy X ray absorptiometry (SXA) and peripheral single-energy X ray absorptiometry (pSXA) are techniques used to measure bone density in the forearm, finger, and heel. Since these screenings do not measure clinically relevant sites, they are not useful for diagnosis of osteoporosis. They *are* useful in assessing the bone density of some elderly people when calcification of bone interferes with the accuracy of DEXA test results.

Ultrasound

The Food and Drug Administration (FDA) recently approved ultrasound devices for bone density readings at the heel or other sites where bones are relatively close to the skin. These ultrasound machines are commonly seen at grocery stores, malls, and health conferences. Ultrasound testing can be helpful in screening for osteoporosis and to predict fracture risk. If you participate in this screening method, you will be asked to put your foot into a machine that takes measurements and provides results in minutes.

Ultrasound measurements are not as precise as DEXA or SXA, but they can predict osteoporosis risk. If your result reveals low bone mass, you will be encouraged to follow up with your doctor, who can order a DEXA scan.

There is a downside to the use of these machines: They measure only the density of the heel bone. Although walking is great exercise, a woman or man who strolls, even for long distances, may have strong bones in their feet but the low impact won't strengthen their hip, back, wrists, arms, and shoulders. A fall can result in a fracture that would not cause a break in a person with healthy bones.

Ronda recently observed one of these testing sessions at an adult center where an eighty-year-old woman with a dowager's hump was told, "Your results are normal." The results of her heel scan, when compared with those of other women her age, may have been in a normal range, but visually her curved upper spine indicated the heel measurement didn't translate to her upper body.

Scoring BMD

Whenever you take a test you get a score. The scoring system for BMD testing isn't the typical 0–100 system. Instead, a reference level is set based on reference levels for optimum bone density for healthy young adults (called a T-score) and for people of your same age and size (called a Z-score). These scores are measured in what statisticians call a standard deviation (SD). This measurement shows the amount of variation from the mean, or average, we would expect to see in a population for some given attribute (in this case, the density of bones). It's an approximation made by sampling a population and making a prediction about that population based on the results. The larger the sample, the more accurate the prediction will be. Standard deviations in bone density are fairly accurate because a large population of men and women have been sampled.

If your BMD score reads 1 SD or more above the average, you are not at risk for osteoporosis—today. If your score is 0 to –1 SD below the average, you will be encouraged to repeat your assessment in a year to see if there are further declines in bone mass. Once your score drops lower, the diagnosis changes. A score between –1 and –2.5 SD (below the average) generates a diagnosis of osteopenia, which means you have already lost at least 10 percent of your bone mass. This is an alert for your doctor who may prescribe medication and lifestyle changes to prevent further bone loss. If your score is more than –2.5 SD (below the average), it tells your doctor you have lost 25 percent or more of your bone mass. You will hear the bad news, "You have osteoporosis." This is when it is mandatory that you begin an active program to prevent further bone loss. With aggressive therapy and a commitment to bone-building exercise, there can even be some new bone growth.

Some facilities that assess BMD look at only the Z-score. If you are active and your score is compared to those of others your age, your Z-score may be high. The sense of security that result can generate may be unwarranted. You still need to know your T-score. Your life depends on it.

T-score	Diagnosis
1.0 to 2.5	No risk of osteoporosis
0.0	Mean
–1.0 to –2.5	Indicates osteopenia
–2.5 or lower	Indicates osteoporosis

Tests That Don't Tell You All You Need to Know
Blood Tests (Serum Blood Levels)

Most people have routine laboratory blood tests as part of their yearly physical. (Have you had yours this year? If not, call your gynecologist or primary physician today to schedule this vital review.) These blood tests are reported to your doctor as serum blood levels. There are many assessments on this routine screen, including serum calcium and phosphorus. In addition, specialized laboratory tests, serum parathyroid hormone (PTH) and vitamin D metabolites, are often added if your medical history reveals a predisposition to osteoporosis.

Although the results of these tests can reveal red flags that signal a need for a DEXA scan, osteoporosis cannot be diagnosed by a blood test.

The level of calcium in your blood does not reflect the density or strength of your bones or how much calcium is in them.

X ray studies

Although it seems logical that an X ray that examines bone would help to establish a diagnosis of osteoporosis, that isn't the case. Approximately 30 to 50 percent of bone mass must be lost before the loss shows up on a routine

X ray. Interestingly, slight overexposure of the X ray film during processing may lead to the appearance of osteoporosis when it is not actually present.

Other Considerations

There is a direct correlation between BMD, as assessed by DEXA, and fracture risk. Bone size must also be considered in the assessment. Males do not have a greater BMD than females, but they do have bigger bones. Similarly, the lower incidence of osteoporosis among African Americans seems to be due to bigger bones rather than greater BMD.

> WARNING: BMD accuracy can be impaired by poorly maintained equipment, patient movement, and coexisting disorders, such as degenerative joint disease.

DEXA studies are also used to monitor the effects of osteoporosis therapy. The precision of measurement is very important in these circumstances. Repeat studies should be conducted at least every two years.

> Medicare will cover the cost for BMD tests every two years, and more frequently if medically necessary, for people at risk. The general medical coverage for BMD, according to the Bone Mass Measurement Act of 1998, includes:
>
> - Estrogen-deficient women at clinical risk for osteoporosis
> - A person with vertebral (spinal) abnormalities demonstrated by X ray to indicate osteoporosis, low bone mass (osteopenia), or vertebral fracture

- A person receiving, or expected to receive, a glucocorticoid therapy equivalent to 7.5 mg or greater of prednisone per day for three months or more
- A person with primary hyperparathyroidism
- A person being monitored to assess a response to FDA-approved osteoporosis drug therapy

WHAT YOU NEED TO KNOW

Eighty percent of low bone mass and osteoporosis goes unnoticed because, until recently, women weren't aware of testing options. *If you have any osteoporosis risk factors, you should ask your health-care provider for a bone density test.* Heel scans, most commonly available to create awareness about this disease, can predict risks, but the DEXA scan is the gold standard for diagnosing osteoporosis. Since many older women already have weak bones, be sure to ask your doctor to assess your risk compared to peak bone mass values in addition to those for women your age. Scoring is based on the results obtained from research on Caucasian women. Nevertheless, it is important for all women to be proactive. Don't panic if your bone density tests demonstrate your bones are as sturdy as a paper kite. New treatments can change the course of this disease.

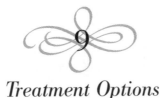

Treatment Options

If your bone scan results in a diagnosis of osteopenia or osteoporosis, your prescribed treatment will be determined by how far your disease has progressed.

- If you have not developed a critically low bone density but are at increased risk for developing osteoporosis, your focus will be on methods to prevent this disease.
- If you have a low bone mass (osteopenia), you will be encouraged to focus on methods of prevention with an emphasis on eliminating as many of the controllable risk factors as possible. (You can't change your gender or genetics.) Medication may also be added to the regimen.
- If a dual-energy X ray absorptiometry (DEXA) scan reveals that you have osteoporosis, your treatment will be designed to prevent further bone loss, increase bone mass, and prevent fractures. This will probably include prescription medication.
- If you already have fractures and deformities, in addition to medication to treat your disease you may also be prescribed drugs and/or treatments to relieve pain caused by fractures.

Stage	Goal
At risk for developing osteoporosis	Prevent bone loss; maintain bone strength
Low bone density but no fractures	Prevent bone loss; increase bone mass; prevent fractures
Low bone density and fractures	Prevent further bone loss; increase bone mass; prevent further fractures; relieve pain
Osteoporosis with disability	Prevent further bone loss; increase bone mass; prevent further fractures; relieve pain; rehabilitate physical capabilities

Gather a group of healthy women over age fifty. Forty percent of them will have undiagnosed osteopenia. Seven percent will have undiagnosed osteoporosis.

Medications for Treatment

Drug interventions currently approved to prevent and treat osteoporosis include estrogen, Selective Estrogen Receptor Modulators (SERMs), bisphosphonates, calcitonin, parathyroid hormone (PHT), and calcium and vitamin D supplements.

Estrogen

Estrogen was the first drug used to treat postmenopausal osteoporosis. Now the FDA supports the use of estrogen to prevent osteoporosis and as part of the management of established osteoporosis.

When estrogen is prescribed for osteoporosis, it is described in two ways:

- Estrogen replacement therapy (ERT) indicates the medication includes only estrogen. It is used only when a woman no longer has a uterus.
- Hormone replacement therapy (HRT) or hormone therapy (HT) is a combination of estrogen and progesterone. It is the drug of choice for postmenopausal women who still have their uterus, because estrogen-only drugs can predispose them to hyperplasia, an abnormal increase (hyper) in the formation of cells (plasia) of the lining of the uterus. Hyperplasia can lead to uterine cancer. The addition of progesterone prevents this condition.

NOTE: In October 2002 the National Institutes for Health (NIH) announced that treatment with estrogen and progesterone (known as HRT) should now be called "hormone therapy" (HT). The new term reflects a more accurate description for the use of these products, which were never intended to be a "replacement" therapy but are a rather useful strategy to treat menopausal symptoms and help maintain bone density.

Estrogen maintains or increases bone mineral density (BMD) by approximately 1 to 3 percent. Although this may seem like a negligible amount, it translates to a significant decrease in osteoporosis fractures. This increase in BMD will occur even when menopause occurred up to ten years earlier, but it is greatest when HRT is started within the first five years after menopause.

Three years of ERT or HRT decreases spinal fractures by 50 to 80 percent and other fractures, including hip and wrist, by approximately 25 percent.

There is a drawback to using estrogen—especially for more than five to ten years. Estrogen increases the risk for breast cancer by up to 30 to 35 percent, so it is contraindicated for any woman who has a family history or any other risk for this disease. ERT and HRT are also contraindicated for women who are predisposed to blood clots in the deep veins of the leg. These kinds of clots can break loose and cause a deadly blockage in the lungs called a pulmonary embolism.

There are many estrogen and estrogen-progesterone combination products available by prescription that are FDA-approved to *prevent* osteoporosis. Only some of them have been approved to *treat* osteoporosis. Estrogen products come in pills and patches, and include:

- Conjugated equine estrogen, 0.625 mg (Premarin®)
- 17 beta-estradiol transdermal patches, 0.05 mg (Estraderm®)
- Transdermal estrogen patch (Vivelle®)

- Piperazine estrone sulfate, 0.75 mg (Ogen®)
- Esterified estrogens, 0.3 mg, 0.625 mg, and 2.5 mg (Estratab®)
- Transdermal estradial (Climara®)
- Estradiol (Estrace®)
- Estropipate (Ortho-Est®)

The estrogen-progesterone products include:

- Estradiol and norethindrone acetate (Activella™)
- Conjugated estrogen with medroxyprogesterone (Femhrt,® Prem-phase,® and Prempro®)

Although many women are using "natural" HRT in the form of pills, patches, and creams that can be purchased without a prescription, there are no studies that show that any of these products prevent bone loss. Most stores, individuals, and Web sites that sell these products cite the benefits of estrogen, but cannot provide any reliable research that shows their specific product does the job when it comes to maintaining or building bone.

Until recently we were sure that estrogen might have a beneficial effect on your heart. New studies show conflicting results. That's why you may hear health professionals say, "The jury is still out" as they continue to weigh the pros and cons of using estrogen. Estrogen is an effective drug for treating osteoporosis. Don't discontinue or refuse it without a conversation with your health-care provider. With the resurgence of compounding pharmacies, you may be able to get a low dose that gives you the benefits you need.

To HRT or Not to HRT? That Is the Question.

In 2002 the National Institutes of Health (NIH) released prelimi-nary results of a study called the Women's Health Initiative (WHI), which followed more than 160,000 postmenopausal women (aver-age age of 63 at the start of the study) who had not had hysterec-tomies (removal of the uterus). Researchers wanted to find out if replacement hormones prevent disease—especially heart disease and osteoporosis—in healthy women without compromising other aspects of their health.

The women were divided into two groups to study the effects of HRT on their health. Half of the women in the study took Prempro,® a drug that combines estrogen with a synthetic progestin (a type of progesterone). The other half did not take HRT.

Although the study was planned to continue for 8.5 years, it was stopped after 5.2 years when the safety committee decided that the benefits of the drug did not offset the risks. The data indicated that during one year, for every 10,000 women taking HRT,

- Eight more women will develop invasive breast cancer
- Seven more women will have a heart attack
- Eight more women will have a stroke
- Eight more women will have blood clots in the lungs
- Eighteen more women will have thromboembolic events

Additionally,

- Six fewer women will have colorectal cancer
- Five fewer women will have hip fractures

The increased breast cancer risk did not appear in the first four years of use. Risk for blood clots was greatest during the first two years of hormone use. The reduced risk for colorectal cancer showed up after three years.

Another group of women taking only estrogen did not show the adverse effects. Their study continues. (Women who have had hysterectomies have no need for progesterone and are typically prescribed estrogen only.)

There is nothing like the results of a just-published research study to generate a lot of confusion. Although the media has made much of this government-funded study, *panic is not justified.* The results did raise concerns for the more than forty million women who are currently menopausal (one-third of whom are taking some form of HRT); however, a woman's personal risk is very small—less than one-tenth of one percent per year.

Women who have been on HRT for more than five years should discuss the results of this study with their doctor, who can help them weigh the risks of continuing their current drug against the benefits it may offer, and determine if using another form of HRT is warranted.

During the 2002 meeting of the National Menopause Society, a panel of prestigious clinicians agreed that HRT and ERT are not warranted solely for the prevention of heart disease since other therapies are available.

If you and your doctor decide that you should stop taking HRT, a cold turkey approach could precipitate a return of menopausal symptoms and withdrawal bleeding. Instead, use a regimen that drops your dose from once a day to every other day for a couple of weeks, then three times a week for several weeks before you stop completely. If bleeding occurs or menopausal symptoms return, you will have to weigh the pros and cons of this medication with your doctor.

NOTE: No segment of the group was separated out as exercisers vs. non-exercisers. Wouldn't it be interesting if only non-exercisers had the increased risk for disease?

Selective Estrogen Receptor Modulators (SERMs)

A class of drugs called Selective Estrogen Receptor Modulators (SERMs), which are not hormones, act like estrogen in many ways. Some people refer to them as "designer estrogens." Raloxifene (Evista® by Lilly & Co.) was introduced in 1997 after it was approved by the FDA to prevent, but not treat, osteoporosis. It is currently the only FDA-approved SERM used to prevent osteoporosis.

New studies show that raloxifene also builds bone, so it is now FDA-approved to treat the disease in postmenopausal women. Using it can reduce the risk of painful vertebral fractures by 40 to 50 percent. Evista® is a drug of choice for women who are at risk for breast cancer, are postmenopausal, and are considered at high risk for developing osteoporosis; however, it is not indicated for women who are predisposed to blood clots. Like most drugs, Evista® has side effects. It has been known to cause leg cramps. A small percentage of women (just over 5 percent) experience hot flashes, although most do not find this bothersome enough to stop taking the drug.

Tamoxifen® is a SERM that reduces the risk of breast cancer recurrence. Doctors have discovered that it also has estrogen-like activity for maintaining bone; however, it is not FDA approved to prevent or treat osteoporosis.

Bisphosphonates

When you get a ring around your bathtub or in your toilet bowl, there are cleaners that magically dissolve this mineral scum. In essence, the chemicals in the cleaner attach themselves to the mineral and make it easy to wash away. Similar chemicals soften hard water and prevent the lime (calcium) deposits that make our porcelain fixtures look so dirty.

These same chemicals, called bisphosphonates, are attracted to calcium. When they are used as a medication, they rush to your bones, bind with the calcium, and powerfully inhibit the work of osteoclasts that resorb bone. This results in a dramatic increase in BMD over time. This, in turn, reduces the incidence of spinal fractures and the potentially devastating fracture of the hip.

Several pharmaceutical companies produce these useful drugs. Each has been the subject of extensive research studies in well-controlled clinical trials regarding their benefits and side effects. Alendronate (Fosamax® by Merck & Co.) was the first bisphosphonate on the market (1997) approved by the FDA to treat osteoporosis in postmenopausal women. Patients with osteoporosis who used the drug showed a 50 percent reducion in the incidence of fracture at the spine, hip, lower arm, and wrist. Women with fractures of their vertebrae who used this drug had fewer days of limited activity. Combined with estrogen, it produces a better effect than either agent alone.

More recently, another bisphosphonate, risedronate (Actonel® by Procter & Gamble Pharmaceuticals and Aventis Pharmaceuticals), was also approved for the treatment of osteoporosis in postmenopausal women. Risedronate increased bone mass, stopped bone loss, produced healthy bone, and reduced the risk of spine and hip fractures by 40 to 50 percent in three to five years. Researchers also observed a rapid, one-year benefit of decreased risk of vertebral fractures.

There is more good news about bisphosphonates. They were originally used only to *treat* osteoporosis. Now they are approved, at a reduced dose and in combination with calcium and vitamin D supplements, to *prevent* osteoporosis in postmenopausal women and in patients whose osteoporosis is steroid induced. They also can be delivered as a weekly dose that will enhance compliance. If you have been on a daily dose of a bisphosphonate, talk to your doctor about this new regimen.

In chapter 6 you learned that there are often unwanted side effects associated with drugs that relieve symptoms or treat a disease. Bisphosphonates have the potential to cause heartburn, painful or difficult swallowing, and gastric reflux—potentially serious erosion of the fragile connection between the esophagus and the stomach.

When these drugs were first released, patients were given very specific instructions about how the drug should be taken. Patients were told, "Take your pill first thing in the morning at least thirty minutes before you eat or drink anything (except water), and remain upright for thirty minutes after you take the medicine." The same instructions applied when the FDA approved a weekly dose. Later studies showed very few gastric problems with these drugs, but the warning as to how to take the medication still applies.

Warnings:

Premenopausal women should be advised about appropriate contraception if bisphosphonates are being considered, since the drug may pose a risk to a fetus.

It is very important to take bisphosphonates as directed to avoid digestive problems.

Anytime you experience discomfort after using any medication you should let your doctor know immediately before making a decision to continue or discontinue using the drug.

Calcitonin

Calcitonin is a hormone made by your thyroid gland. It monitors the amount of calcium in your blood. If blood calcium levels get high, calcitonin activity will decrease the number and activity of the osteoclasts. That prevents calcium from leaving the bone and returns calcium already in the blood to the bone. The result is increased bone mass.

When researchers are looking for new ways to treat disease, they often look to animals to find out if they have the same biochemical processes as humans. That research has revealed that many animals have calcitonin. Further investigation revealed that salmon calcitonin was the best variety to use to treat osteoporosis. Now pharmacological preparations of both synthetic human and salmon calcitonin are available, but only salmon calcitonin has been FDA-approved for osteoporosis treatment.

Calcitonin, in combination with a calcium and vitamin D supplement, is a useful osteoporosis treatment for women who are more than five years postmenopause, have a low BMD, and are not candidates for estrogen treatment. It is available for injection (Calcimar® by Rhone-Poulenc Rorer), or as the more popular nasal spray (Miacalcin® by Sandoz), which is rapidly absorbed through the tissues in your nose. Patients who have difficulty swallowing pills prefer this drug. Calcitonin can reduce the risk of spinal fractures by 40 percent, but it doesn't work as well on other bones. Another advantage of this drug is that it also relieves the pain of acute spinal fractures.

Salmon calcitonin is one of the safest drugs available for the treatment of osteoporosis. Drawbacks are a runny nose and, for some, occasional nasal bleeding caused by drug irritation.

Parathyroid Hormone

Our bodies make many hormones besides estrogen and testosterone. One of these is parathyroid hormone (PTH), which is produced by four pea-sized parathyroid glands located near, but unrelated to, the thyroid. The sole purpose of the parathyroid glands is to keep the calcium levels in the blood in a very tight range. By doing this, they also control how much calcium is in bone. When blood calcium levels are low, PTH can stimulate the production of osteoblasts. Researchers have long believed that PTH could be an impressive treatment for osteoporosis.

In November 2002 the FDA approved the use of a synthetic form of PTH to treat osteoporosis in men and postmenopausal women who are at high risk for a fracture. Teriparatide (Forteo® by Lilly) is supplied in a disposable pen device that can be used for up to twenty-eight days to give daily self-administered injections. Research showed that a 20 mg daily dose can reduce the risk of spinal fractures by 65 percent and other fractures by 53 percent. All patients who used the drug had an increase in bone density.

Unlike other therapies that slow the breakdown of bone, teriparatide increases the number and action of bone-building osteoblasts. Additionally, no increase was seen in fracture risk for at least eighteen months after treatment ended and significant drug interactions were not observed. The drug is not recommended for children, adolescents, or people who have another bone disease called Paget's disease.

Although a daily, self-administered injection may seem drastic, the bone mass gains are worthwhile for men and women who are at risk for a fracture that could be life threatening.

Calcium

It is now common knowledge that calcium supplements can help prevent osteoporosis. We still don't know how effective these supplements are in osteoporosis treatment. The effects of calcium on fracture rates have been inconsistent. Regardless, calcium supplements are now a routine adjunct to any drug used to treat osteoporosis, and most doctors who must prescribe drugs that can weaken bones encourage their patients to take a calcium supplement.

We believe that all women should eat foods rich in calcium *and* take a calcium supplement. In chapter 13 you will learn much more about this important mineral that is so integral to bone health, as well as the variety of calcium supplements available, absorption issues, foods that are rich in calcium, and the drugs and foods that interact with calcium to prevent adequate absorption. Until then, know this:

- Your calcium supplement will, of necessity, be combined with another compound that keeps it stabilized. The most common supplements are calcium carbonate, calcium lactate, calcium citrate, and calcium gluconate. Your choice will depend on how well you tolerate the supplement (some supplements give some people gas) and your budget (expensive products are not necessarily better).

- Your body cannot absorb more than 500 mg of calcium at a time. The amount of calcium a compound yields is called its elemental calcium. Check this important number on the bottles of the supplements you are considering.

- Choose reliable products that have the USP symbol on the label. This assures that the supplement has been tested and will dissolve properly in your body.

- There's no benefit in using a "natural" supplement. Unless it is USP-labeled, a supplement from oyster shell, dolomite, or bonemeal may be contaminated with ingredients that are unsafe.

- Whenever possible, take your calcium supplement with dairy foods to enhance absorption.

- Calcium supplements (and dairy products) interact with some prescription drugs. This can make the drug less effective. You can resolve this problem by taking your calcium supplement two hours before or after those medications. Drug classes affected by this phenomenon are listed in chapter 13.

Calcium supplements interact with some foods that bind the calcium in a way that prevents absorption. A list of these foods appears in chapter 13.

Emerging Treatments

Several new therapies are being studied for the prevention and treatment of osteoporosis. They include other SERMs, bisphosphonates, fluoride, statin drugs, and non-loop diuretics.

Now that SERMs and bisphosphonates are proven osteoporosis treatments, other versions of these drugs are being studied in an attempt to discover if they are as effective as those that are already on the market. There is also research in New Zealand using zoledronic acid (Zometa® by Novartis Pharmaceuticals), a bisphosphonate that can be given intravenously. Preliminary results show that an annual infusion of the drug resulted in the same effects as those achieved with oral doses of a bisphosphonate. Taking a drug as instructed is what makes it work. Nevertheless, most patients inadvertently forget a dose now and then. Look into the future: Wouldn't it be wonderful if osteoporosis could be treated once a year during your annual trip to the doctor for a mammogram, Pap smear, and other routine tests?

Fluoride

When you hear the word fluoride, you probably think of teeth. You should also think of bones. Health sleuths are always observing the changes that occur when a chemical is used in any situation. In the case of fluoride, a lower incidence of osteoporosis in areas where there was fluoride in the water made scientists sit up and take notice. A well-planned research study revealed that people who drink fluoridated water have a higher bone density than those who don't. This increase occurs mostly in trabecular and some cortical bone. As is often the case with research, researchers still haven't ferreted out the hows and whys of the change. They are unclear about the quality of that new bone, which in some studies wasn't very strong. Regardless, it's an important finding.

The studies regarding the success of fluoride have been dramatic but small. Several combinations of slow-release fluoride and calcium citrate are being used in Europe, but the jury is still out in the United States, where fluoride has not been approved to treat osteoporosis.

Statins

Millions of Americans are now taking cholesterol-lowering drugs known as statins. Doctors who continue to monitor the progress of postmenopausal women who use these drugs have discovered that their patients appear to have a lower risk of osteoporosis-related fractures. There aren't enough data yet to warrant the use of these drugs to prevent or treat osteoporosis, but it's rewarding when drugs have *positive* side effects.

Non-Loop Diuretics

Another study showed that hydrochlothiazide (a common diuretic not in the category of loop diuretics that can cause bone loss) preserves bone density at the hip and spine over a three-year period when compared to a placebo. The benefit, though modest, makes this drug a consideration in programs to prevent osteoporosis—especially in women who need to take diuretics.

The aggressive research currently being conducted seems certain to provide additional effective drugs to prevent or end bone loss or to rebuild bone. We are indeed encouraged that our premise—living long can mean living well—is a reality for smart women everywhere.

Herbs, Soy, and Supplements

There is worldwide use of herbal and homeopathic products, in addition to prescription drugs, to treat a variety of medical conditions, including osteoporosis. Our audiences tell us they look to these "natural" healing, alternative, or complementary therapies in a quest for control of their health—especially when they believe the medical system is unresponsive to their needs.

According to the Institute for Safe Medication Practices, only about half the patients who use complementary or alternative strategies will tell their doctors what they are doing for fear of criticism. It would be arrogant of us to deny the efficacy of a variety of healing traditions, including those that are alternatives to Western standards.

When it comes to herbs, your pharmacist remains a reliable resource for authoritative information backed by scientific references. If he or she doesn't know an answer, your best resources are *The Honest Herbal* by Varro E. Tyler, Ph.D., and *The American Pharmaceutical Association Practical Guide to Natural Medicines* by Andrea Peirce. Both books tell what, if any, valid research has been conducted on common herbs as well as the assets and liabilities of using them.

Soy and Phytoestrogens

Phytoestrogen is the term used for estrogens that come from plant sources. Phytoestrogens are believed to be a safe strategy for women who cannot or do not want to take estrogen for relief of menopausal symptoms, such as hot flashes. Researchers at the University of Illinois who studied the effects of soy discovered that postmenopausal women who were on a high-soy diet for six months had a slight increase in (only) spinal bone density; however, the researchers agreed that additional long-term studies are needed to explore this prospective benefits of soy.

Soy protein contains compounds known as isoflavones. Studies in Japan and Italy, in and out of laboratories, focused on ipriflavone, a synthetic isoflavone. These early studies suggested that an ipriflavone supplement prevents bone loss and might increase bone mass. A more recent clinical double-blind study (in which neither the patient nor the doctor knew if the pill given to the patient was the medicine or a placebo) revealed that ipriflavone was no more effective than a placebo.

Science is an evolutionary process. Conclusions derived from a single study or two should always be viewed as preliminary. It remains to be seen whether additional investigation will affirm or deny that supplemental phytoestrogen in the form of soy or ipriflavone pills is useful to prevent or treat osteoporosis. In the United States there is no control over the marketing of supplements. Although many companies promote ipriflavone supplements for bone health, they are not an FDA-supported treatment strategy. Like many other prescription and nonprescription options, this supplement has a downside. All studies showed that *some* of the women taking ipriflavone developed lymphocytopenia, a condition marked by an abnormally low level of disease-fighting white blood cells (lymphocytes). This side effect does not occur when soy is the source of the isoflavone.

Soy is a viable alternative to meat. It's high in fiber and cholesterol free, and doesn't contain the antibiotics and hormones that are of concern to folks who want to eat foods without additives. We are advocates for the use of food over supplements to get the nutrients you need. Meanwhile, we agree with investigators who discourage the use of ipriflavone, saying it isn't a safe or effective treatment for osteoporosis and should be discouraged until further studies affirm or revoke this position.

Neither of the following is recommended to treat osteoporosis:

- Injectable growth hormone is beneficial for bone development in calcium-deficient children and adults but has harmful side effects.
- Anabolic steroids also promote bone formation, but their use by women is limited by their virilizing effects (and by men because of the harmful effects on the cardiovascular system and prostate).

Treating the Pain of Osteoporosis

Patients who experience osteoporosis-based fractures often endure considerable pain. Some of that pain diminishes or disappears as the fracture heals. For many people, the pain becomes chronic. Narcotics and other drugs, available by prescription only, provide relief for acute pain, but they can produce tolerance and have many side effects (including constipation, which is most common). These drugs are suitable for short-term use only. Aspirin, acetaminophen, or any over-the-counter, nonsteroid anti-inflammatory drugs (NSAIDs—e.g., naproxen, ibuprofen) are the safest choices, although in some patients their side effects with long-term use or overuse are gastric irritation and bleeding.

In addition to treating the pain of osteoporotic fractures with over-the-counter and prescription drugs, other strategies that are often part of multi-disciplinary treatment options include the following:

- Physical therapy in which a trained professional suggests an appropriate range of movements to improve muscle strength and flexibility. Activities are designed to keep patients active, prevent falls, and release the body's natural painkilling endorphins.
- Heat in the form of warm showers and microwave-heated packs (including air-activated wearable heat wraps), and/or cold in the form of cold packs, bags of frozen peas, and ice packs.
- Transcutaneous Electrical Nerve Stimulation (TENS) units, which are small machines that use mild electrical current to block the path of pain signals from the source of the injury to the brain.
- Massage therapy, which relaxes stiff muscles caused by pain. Osteoporosis patients should avoid deep-muscle massage in favor of the circular or rhythmic motion known as Swedish massage.

- Acupuncture, a technique that has been used successfully in China for thousands of years to reduce pain, and that is widely available today. It is administered by a licensed practitioner who uses thin, presterilized, disposable needles to stimulate pathways that release neurochemicals from the brain and other tissues. This contributes to the reduction of pain and inflammation.

- Acupressure, which provides pressure over areas called trigger points to help relieve pain. Pressure should never be applied near the spine in patients with fragile osteoporotic bones.

- Braces, which relieve pain by stabilizing and supporting joints near a fracture. They allow patients to remain active while a fracture heals. Braces are most often used during the healing phase of a spinal fracture.

- Exercise, which encourages movement of stiff muscles and keeps a patient mobile, should be done at a level a patient can tolerate. (See chapter 10.)

- Psychologically oriented or mind/body methods of pain relief, which make use of the powerful connection between our physical well-being and our thoughts, feelings, and behaviors. Double-blind, peer-reviewed studies published in reputable journals reveal we can train our mind to consciously and unconsciously change our body's response to pain. Some effective tension-relief strategies are progressive relaxation, rhythmic breathing, hypnosis, and biofeedback, as well as visual imagery, affirmations, and therapy. These activities help patients deal with the stress and depression that can accompany osteoporosis. There is no single strategy that works better than another, and each person may be more comfortable with some than with others.

Any of the preceding approaches will often be combined with anti-depressant drugs to manage the chronic pain of osteoporotic fractures. Tricyclic Antidepressants (TCAs) and Selective Serotonin Reuptake Inhibitors (SSRIs) increase various brain chemicals and restore a feeling of well-being. Low doses are usually effective in giving patients with pain an edge in preventing further physical deterioration and regaining an active life.

> Maintaining BMD is nearly as effective as increasing BMD in reducing fracture risks.

WHAT YOU NEED TO KNOW

There are now many types of medication available to treat osteoporosis. Unless you have a personal or family history of breast cancer, your doctor may recommend a drug combination of estrogen and progesterone. If you have had your uterus removed, you don't need the progesterone. "Designer estrogens" known as SERMs (Evista®) are one of the alternatives to estrogen for women who are at risk for breast cancer. The bisphosphonates (such as Fosamax® and Actonel®) and calcitonin (Miacalcin®) stop or slow bone breakdown, prevent bone loss, and actually increase bone mass in women with osteoporosis. PTH (Forteo®)

increases bone mass by stimulating the number and action of cells that build bone.

Don't fall into the trap of believing that because you are taking a prescription to maintain or increase bone mass you don't need to continue taking a calcium and vitamin D supplement and eating a high-calcium diet. Continuing to do both assures optimal treatment results.

If you are diagnosed with osteoporosis, you need to discuss these treatment options with your doctor, pay attention to your body's response to the choices made, and stick with the regimen that is the best fit for managing your disease and improving your bone health. Since failure to comply with doctors' orders can have serious consequences, it is imperative to develop a routine that assures you take your medicine exactly as prescribed.

If you experience chronic pain, ask your health-care providers for suggestions to get relief. Stick with your program. Persistence and patience are the keys to successfully treating this disease. Improvement can occur. Even if you can't replace all your lost bone, every millimeter of increased bone density is a big step toward a healthy future.

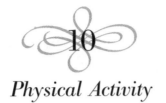

Physical Activity

Suppose, after reading this book, you have a DEXA scan that reveals you have osteopenia or osteoporosis. Or, in a worst-case scenario, you have a simple fall that results in a not-so-simple fracture. Perhaps, like too many of our older friends, a simple movement causes such severe back pain that you call your doctor, who orders X rays that show you have one or more spontaneous fractures in your spine. Maybe you have already been diagnosed with osteopenia or osteoporosis and picked up this book to get the latest updates on self-care. Regardless, the treatment your doctor outlines for you will take into consideration all the factors outlined in earlier chapters of this book. Whether that regimen includes estrogen, SERMs, bisphosphonates, calcitonin, parathyroid hormone, or supplements, you can pretty much count on a recommendation to exercise. If your diagnosis was precipitated by a fracture, your doctor will probably send you to a physical therapist first for evaluation, to see whether you can safely practice exercise. If so, you will get an introductory program there and, on discharge, be given instructions on flexibility, coordination, and balance, and how to continue building muscle and bone strength. If you already have an exercise strategy in place, it may or may not need to be modified to support the changes in bone density provided by exercise. And if exercise has not been a part of your lifestyle, the instruction to exercise may have little meaning for you. How do you begin? What's the best kind?

Exercise, for the purpose of treating osteoporosis, includes three kinds of activities:

1. Aerobic exercise on a hard surface to strengthen bone using impact
2. Anaerobic exercise that strengthens muscle and attached bone using force
3. Movement that improves coordination, balance, and flexibility

Aerobic Exercise

The word "aerobic" means "with oxygen." From the perspective of exercise physiology, aerobic exercise is an activity that requires the presence of oxygen in the muscle cell in order to convert stored fat (energy) to fuel for muscle work. For the purpose of treating bones, your aerobic activity must cause what physiologists call a strike force—your foot must strike the floor with force. That impact moves through your feet, up your legs, and into your hips and lower back, strengthening those supporting bones. Weight-bearing aerobic exercise uses the big muscles of your lower body for a sufficient amount of time—and often enough—to gain benefits in all systems of your body, including your skeletal system (your bones).

In addition to strike force or impact, your effort must be intense enough to force your heart and lungs to work harder than normal but not so hard that you get out of breath. That includes activities such as fitness walking, dancing, kickboxing, step aerobics, jogging, skating—

anything you do on your feet. Although exercises like cycling and swimming can make you aerobically fit, they do nothing for your bones because you are not bearing weight.

To gain the benefits of aerobic exercise, you must do your activity at least five days a week until you are aerobically fit. Then a three- or four-day-a-week regimen will help you sustain that level of fitness and ensure that you are always contributing to bone health. You'll learn more about aerobic exercise principles in chapter 14.

Anaerobic Exercise

Another type of exercise important to bones is anaerobic (without oxygen) exercise. Unlike aerobic exercise, which primarily uses fat for fuel and requires oxygen to convert the fat to energy, anaerobic exercise primarily uses stored sugar (glucose) to fuel a muscle and requires little, if any oxygen. That may sound silly, because you never stop breathing and inhaling oxygen when you exercise. But when you do an exercise that challenges a muscle so intensely that you can't deliver enough oxygen to burn fat for fuel, the muscle calls on that alternative glucose-burning system. If you get breathless or "feel the burn," you are exercising anaerobically.

Anaerobic exercise is designed to tire one or more muscle groups. It is training for strength and endurance. You may also hear it described as resistance training, weight training, or bodybuilding. It's also called weight bearing because you are using weights or resistance to make muscles stronger and denser. Since the muscle is pulling on the bone to which it is attached, as the muscle gets stronger and denser, the bone gets stronger, too.

You need to strength train at least two non-consecutive days a week. Spend five to ten minutes on upper body work using commercial weights (or tin cans or jugs of water) or the weight of your body (push-ups or modified push-ups), and five to ten minutes on lower body work using machine weights or the weight of your lower body (squats and lunges). Your goal for strength training the lower body is to be able to get up from a chair without using your arms to give you an added push. You'll learn more about the principles of anaerobic exercise in chapter 14.

A small group of postmenopausal women who wore a weighted vest during a five-year exercise program directed by Christine Snow, Ph.D., Director of the Bone Research Laboratory at Oregon State University, maintained or increased bone density in all regions of the hip when compared to a control group of exercisers who were active but did not use the weighted vest. The participants met three times a week for one-hour sessions that included a walking and stretching warm-up and cool-down and an activity session that included lower body resistance training and aerobic stepping and/or jumping for fitness. Two women in the program reversed their osteoporosis.

Beyond Weight Bearing and Bearing Weight

There's an often-overlooked dimension of fitness that is particularly important to people who want to prevent falls. Since the emphasis isn't on conditioning bones or muscles in the traditional sense, these activities that improve balance, coordination, and flexibility are sometimes called the "softer" side of fitness. Nothing could be further from the truth. People who practice these disciplines are strong and centered. If you want a balanced fitness program, introduce yourself to yoga, tai chi, Pilates, or any of the martial arts. The benefits gained using these disciplines are in direct proportion to the amount of time you invest in practicing them. More is better.

If you aren't a fitness buff, it's not too late to start exercising. Whether you are young or not so young, you'll experience gains. Because exercise benefits cannot be stored, the axiom "use it or lose it" applies here. If you have been exercising but your program has been non–weight bearing, or if you do only one kind of aerobic exercise, consider broadening your perspective. Cross-training is a healthy way to keep fit. If you square dance aerobically on Monday, Wednesday, and Friday and fitness walk on Tuesday and Thursday, you are cross-training. On the days you focus on anaerobic fitness, cut back on the amount of time you practice aerobic fitness. If you spend forty to fifty minutes a day on your fitness health, you will set the stage for long-term health and wellness.

In chapter 14 you will read more about the principles of exercise that keep people motivated, and learn the five steps that can help you start and maintain a lifetime habit that can outwit osteoporosis.

WHAT YOU NEED TO KNOW

Any sound strategy to combat osteoporosis should begin with a solid aerobics program that focuses on weight-bearing exercises like fitness walking, dancing, kickboxing, step aerobics, jogging, or skating. In addition, you should engage in an anaerobic strength-building program (lifting weights) for both the upper and lower body to increase bone strength, and add movement that will improve your balance, coordination, and flexibility. A cross-training program encourages all-over fitness.

It takes time to get and stay bone-fit. The results are worth it.

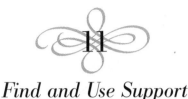

Find and Use Support

"Just do it." It's easier said than done. In fact, keeping motivated is one of the toughest dilemmas for people who choose to alter their life. So what can we offer you to help you stick with it?

If success breeds success, looking at what has worked for others is a place to start. For more than seventy years, the support groups of twelve-step recovery programs have been a force behind life changes for people whose lives were perilously threatened by addictions to substances (e.g., drugs, alcohol, food) or behaviors (e.g., gambling, shopping, relationships). The twelve-step model has been adapted so widely that there are now support groups for almost anything. Successful weight loss, also formerly a "just do it" industry, now uses coaching and support to enhance success. Why do these popular support programs work?

Anytime you make an adjustment in your lifestyle, there's a shift in the rhythm of your life. Unless the rewards are great, constant vigilance is required to stay the course.

Taking a vitamin or prescription drug takes seconds and is a change that is easily adopted. That's not the case when it comes to time-consuming exercise and dietary changes. Your changes also affect the people with whom you live and work. Even if they support your choice to make your life healthier, they are unlikely to be eager to make the shifts in *their* lives required to truly support you. Additionally, a diagnosis of osteoporosis and the warnings that a risk for fracture is significant are stunning developments in the lives of most women. They look to others for the wisdom of their experience and the cheerleading. You can do it!

Support Groups

There are support groups springing up nationwide for people with osteoporosis. You can gather with people who share your disease and help problem-solve any dilemma that may rear its ugly head. Typically, a support group will invite guest speakers, distribute educational materials, and share gossip regarding which doctors and treatments give good results. The best resource is your local osteoporosis center or the office of a physician whose treatment specialty includes osteoporosis. The National Osteoporosis Foundation has a nationwide network of support groups called Building Strength Together. It also provides guidelines to help start a group. The foundation's contact number and Web site address can be found in the Resources section at the end of this book.

Internet

The Internet is a rich resource for learning more about osteoporosis, medications that treat the disease, and exercise programming.

Use a search engine and type in the word "osteoporosis," the name of your osteoporosis medication, or the word "exercise." If you use the Internet frequently, you probably have a favorite search engine, but because each one lists different resources, try several for more results. There are also chat groups and newsgroups where you can meet people who share your interest in osteoporosis and who can give you immediate feedback and support. Your Internet provider should have an extensive list of chat groups. Our search on the Internet also located individual Web sites created by people who have their own resource lists for learning more about osteoporosis.

These resources come with a caveat: "User beware." Although there are many reputable people, agencies, and associations willing to help you, there are also unscrupulous people who may give you false information or attempt to sell you something that may not be useful or wise for you to use. The Internet can be a great resource for value when it comes to buying supplements or prescriptions, but remember, these drugs can react with other supplements and prescriptions. If you are on a prescription drug, you shouldn't add anything to your regimen without checking with your doctor. Your pharmacist can also discuss drug interactions with you.

Psychological Support

The psychological issues that can emerge when you or someone in your family has the chronic pain of osteoporosis fractures can be overwhelming. Sure, you can sweat it out on your own and pull yourself up by the bootstraps, or you can yield, admit you aren't coping as well as you had hoped, and get some professional help. If your disease challenges your mental health, don't fail to seek counseling. The coping skills and attitude adjustments that result from the wise counsel of professionals are well worth your time and money. Always interview a prospective mental health professional with the same care you would take to interview a specialist of any kind. Pay attention to gut feelings about the person as well as to the setting where the counseling is offered. Ask others in the same boat if they can give you the name of a professional they know and trust. The acknowledgment that psychological strategies can support the prevention and treatment of disease is one of the great breakthroughs in the medical profession. Take advantage of it.

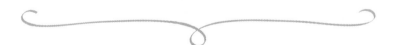

WHAT YOU NEED TO KNOW

One factor highly correlated with successful change is good support. Typically this involves family and friends, but it can extend to professional assistance or peer-related groups and support agencies, including those that focus on helping people with osteoporosis.

When you make a mutual commitment to others to give and receive support, you will find the encouragement, education, and understanding to help you through the many rough spots you may encounter in the treatment of your bone health.

Section IV

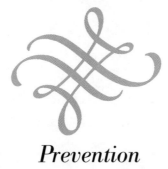

Prevention

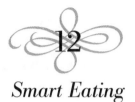

Smart Eating

Osteoporosis is preventable. Science continues to identify causes and improve methods for diagnosis and treatment. We can say, unequivocally, that the ravages of this devastating disease—brittle bones, unnecessary fractures, and dowager's humps—can be tempered in our lifetime and eliminated in future generations if we optimize bone health throughout life. This can be accomplished with changes in lifestyle that improve not only bone strength but other important health parameters as well.

Proper Diet

Americans, especially women, are manic about their diet. They combine foods, count calories, manipulate nutrients, buy diet books, deprive themselves, and pay outrageous prices for pills and potions, hoping that the "right" diet will bring them the slim look and/or healthy body they crave. This penchant for dieting can have detrimental effects on bone, especially if there are other predisposing factors for osteoporosis.

The solution to dieting is simple. Instead of focusing on diet for weight loss, begin thinking of "diet" in the context provided in most dictionaries: a way of choosing foods. Join the mainstream and eat "naturally." Choose a calorie-sufficient diet that is low in fat, low in sugar (especially added sugar), high in fiber, balanced, and varied. If you follow a diet that meets dietary guidelines for the milk group, you will get nutrients that can prevent osteoporosis. A calcium supplement provides additional insurance. (See chapters 9 and 13.) In the same way that a good foundation in a building sets the stage for the structure over it, a good diet is the foundation for health if you plan to live well for a long time.

There is growing evidence of a positive link between fruit and vegetable intake and bone health. Recent findings in a Tufts University study of 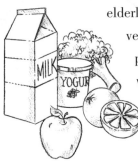 elderly people showed that men who ate more fruits and vegetables and less candy had stronger bones than peers who indulged in sweet treats. Remarkably, it was even true when the fruit and vegetable eaters had less calcium in their diet. This suggests that other nutrients besides calcium contribute to stronger bones. Although the difference in women's groups in the study wasn't as significant, it is believed that a diet with fewer empty calories plays a more significant role in osteoporosis prevention than we had thought. Fruits and vegetables are rich in potassium, magnesium, beta-carotene, fiber, and vitamin D—dietary elements that facilitate the environment in which bones thrive.

Dietary Calcium

It is so important that we will say it again: A diet low in calcium, at any age, is a shortcut to unhealthy bones. Calcium is the most abundant mineral in the body. About 99 percent of it is stored in your bones. It makes up three pounds of normal body weight. It does more than support the growth of healthy bones. It is also essential for blood clotting, nerve transmission, and muscle contraction. In short, the importance of calcium begins at birth and continues throughout life. Think about it: When we attempt to feed starving children, the first line of defense is often powdered milk, which is high in protein and calcium. Without milk in the formative years, bones can't reach maximum density. Adding a high-calcium diet later in life can improve bone mineral content and slow bone loss, but by then it is too late to prevent osteoporosis.

Despite what vitamin salespeople tell you, the best-absorbed source of calcium comes from milk and milk products. If you choose low-fat or non-fat milk, you get the added benefit of a product that is lower in fat.

Which Milk Will You Choose?

Milk Type	Calories/8 oz.	mg CA*/8 oz.	gm fat/8 oz.
whole	150	~300	8
2 percent	121	~300	4
1 percent	102	~300	2
nonfat	80	~325	0

*CA is the abbreviation for calcium
NOTE: Some stores carry calcium-fortified milk.

Although the U.S. dairy group uses athletes, models, and performers in the popular "Got Milk?" newspaper and magazine ads, a U.S. Agriculture Department study of American girls aged twelve through nineteen found that as the girls got older they drank more diet and sugar-filled soda and less milk. Teens who drank the most milk lived in families in which their parents were milk drinkers. Parents *can* set an example for a disease-free lifestyle.

About Milk-Free Diets

People who are proponents of a milk-free diet (what will their bones be like when they are old?) make logical but ridiculous statements, including, "Humans are the only species that continue to drink milk after they are weaned." Humans are also the only species that gets osteoporosis. You will also hear, "Dark green, leafy vegetables are an excellent source of calcium." Once again that is only part of the story. Calcium is not as well absorbed from these foods as it is from milk or milk products. Remember, the vitamin D in milk products, which makes calcium more absorbable, isn't present in vegetables. Most of these "you don't need milk" proponents neglect to add that it takes 1-1/2 cups of kale, 3 cups of broccoli, or 10 cups of cabbage to get the amount of calcium found in one glass of milk, 2/3 cup of yogurt, or 1/2 cup of cottage cheese. If you can eat five cups of greens a day, go for it.

We are such strong advocates for milk in the diet that you may think we work for the Dairy Council. We don't; we just prefer the milk-mustache route.

> If you are premenopausal, you need at least 1,000 mg of calcium a day.
>
> If you are postmenopausal, you need at least 1,200 to 1,500 mg of calcium a day.

Lactose Intolerance

Some people develop an intolerance to the milk sugar, lactose. As they get older, their bodies no longer produce lactase, the enzyme that breaks down milk sugar to glucose. Instead, the undigested lactose is eaten in the intestine by bacteria that live there naturally. The gassy waste products produced by the bacteria that process the lactose can create uncomfortable abdominal cramping. If you are lactose intolerant, you may still be able to eat calcium-containing milk products, including yogurt, buttermilk, or sour cream. (There are naturally occurring bacteria in these products that break lactose apart.) There is also an over-the-counter product, Lactaid,® which does what a lactase-deficient digestive system cannot. If neither of these strategies works, get a referral from your doctor to meet with a dietitian, who can provide guidelines for managing a diet that is deficient in calcium, riboflavin, vitamin D, and protein.

There are approximately 300 mg of calcium in:

Milk

1/2 cup powdered milk

1 cup milk (nonfat, 1%, 2%, whole)

Cheese

1-1/2 oz. cheddar-type cheese

2-1/2 oz. American (processed) cheese

1-3/4 oz. mozzarella (part nonfat milk) cheese

Other Dairy Products

6 oz. low-fat plain yogurt

1 cup low-fat fruited yogurt

1 cup pudding made with milk

1-3/4 cups ice cream or ice milk

Fish

5 oz. salmon, with bone

7 sardines, with bone

2 cups shrimp

Vegetables

1-1/2 cups cooked spinach

2 cups collard greens

3 cups broccoli

10 cups raw cabbage

2-1/2 cups rhubarb

Calcium-fortified foods include:

bread	orange juice	cranberry juice
ready-to-eat cereals	milk	

Caffeine in Your Diet

The jury is still out. Does caffeine increase bone loss or not? Our research for this book revealed that there is no consensus on this question, because the scientific literature is conflicting. Recent data don't support the long-held belief that caffeine is bad for you. If you have been diagnosed with thin bones, take the high road. Don't wait for the scientists to come to a clear conclusion. Caffeine is an addictive drug. Those of us who start our day with a race to the local coffee merchant for a latte or to our neighborhood market for a caffeine-filled Diet Coke® know that caffeine gives our morning a jump start. The best advice, especially when you've been told you have fragile bones, is to limit caffeine intake to a couple of cups (or cans) a day. Don't try to remove caffeine from your diet without a slow tapering-off period, or you may experience throbbing headaches or other symptoms of withdrawal.

Alcohol in Your Diet

Alcohol has been shown to increase the excretion of calcium. Yes, we know a glass or two of red wine a day is good for heart health. But more than two glasses a day may be too much if you have or are predisposed to osteoporosis. Consider limiting yourself to one or two drinks a week or as a treat on special occasions.

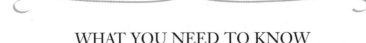

WHAT YOU NEED TO KNOW

You are receiving plenty of encouragement from many professionals to maintain a healthy weight. The bottom line, if you will excuse the pun, is that an appropriate diet for someone who has or could get osteoporosis doesn't come with some of the typical "lose weight" dietary advice the media perpetuates. Writers and reporters are savvy about your desire to learn how to improve your health. That's why there are so many health-oriented, attention-getting headlines. Some are misleading. When you hear or read about diet strategies for quick weight loss, think long term. If healthy eating (and exercise) in your younger years can prevent most diseases of longevity, why not take out an insurance policy now? Instead of eating for results that will supposedly make you look good at your high school reunion, that wedding, or the beach, begin today to eat for your life.

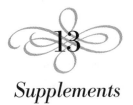

Supplements

Finally, we get to supplements. Two of our most frequently asked questions are "What should I take?" and "What is the correct dosage?" Thanks to ads, infomercials, famous personalities, and neighbors telling you to take this or take that, especially if they are selling a high-profit item, consumers remain confused.

The supplement market, which exploded when shrewd entrepreneurs scurried to take advantage of sloppy 1994 legislation, can bewilder the most savvy health professionals. Suddenly, labels for vitamin, mineral, herbal, hormone, and amino acid products promised cures for and relief from every symptom imaginable. Supplements are sold without the Food and Drug Administration (FDA) approval that regulates prescription drugs. The Federal Trade Commission (FTC) stepped in with guidelines to assure that advertising stays truthful and substantiated, but only a few players in the industry are abiding by those rules.

A Hungry Body
Your body craves many vitamins and minerals every day. These micro-nutrients don't have calories, but without them, you can't digest, absorb, or metabolize the calories you eat. Vitamins and minerals help your body heal

injuries, fight disease, and drive the thousands of chemical reactions taking place in your body every second. If you are like most Americans, you are whipping out your wallet and jumping on the supplement bandwagon in an effort to improve your health. Some of you may be carrying a good thing too far by taking many different supplements every day. It's not necessary.

Some of the most exciting developments in the field of nutrition are the new discoveries that identify previously unknown and life-essential substances in food. With each discovery, a new group of pills is sure to be produced as entrepreneurs take their piece of the supplement pie. Remember our first rule of thumb: *Supplements are not a substitute for food.* You are better off using the dietary recommendations in chapter 12. Go for foods that provide balance, variety, and sufficient calories, and foods that are lower in sugar and fat and higher in fiber. Think food first, then supplements.

Don't get us wrong. We are strong proponents of supplementation in general—especially when it comes to calcium and vitamin D, which can prevent osteoporosis. But don't go overboard.

Calcium

Whether you are five, twenty-five, fifty-five, or eighty-five years young, the amount of calcium in your diet affects the density and strength of your bones now and in the future. Calcium is the most abundant mineral in your body, and 99 percent of it is stored in your bones. But it's the "nonbone" functions of calcium that are critical to your bones' ability to retain stored calcium. Muscle contraction, blood clotting, the body's self-defense mechanism to fight infection, and even calcium's role in every living cell all compete for dietary calcium on a daily basis.

Milk, milk products, fish with bones (canned sardines and canned salmon), and green leafy vegetables are the primary and best sources of dietary calcium. If you eat enough of these foods, you will meet your calcium needs. Since many women don't, insurance in the form of a calcium supplement is wise.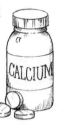

So which calcium supplement is best? First of all, beware of the word "natural." Marketing experts remind supplement entrepreneurs that if they put the word "natural" in front of a product name, their customers will pay up to three times more than they would for the identical product without the "natural" moniker. Germs are natural. Disease is natural. Bee stings are natural. Snakebites are natural. We don't want them and neither do you. "Natural" may be the most overused word in the health-promotion field today. Calcium sold in the form of dolomite, bonemeal, or crushed oyster shells is often sold with the "natural" label, but some of these calcium sources are filled with lead or other toxic materials. How's that for natural?

Instead of natural products, use a laboratory-produced calcium. There are several. Each is composed of calcium combined with another compound to make it stable. The amount of calcium that is released from the compound and absorbed in your body is dependent on the chemical composition of that compound. That is why, when you purchase a supplement, you need to know how much *elemental calcium* the tablet delivers. This information is on the bottle.

Calcium carbonate is the most popular calcium supplement because it is so inexpensive and it is concentrated; you need only two or three tablets to meet recommended daily allowances of 1,200 to 1,500 mg of calcium per day. Since many antacids contain calcium carbonate, they are often recommended for calcium supplementation. But beware: If the antacid also contains aluminum, the calcium will not be absorbed.

Tums® is the best known of the inexpensive, non-aluminum, non-magnesium, calcium carbonate–containing antacids. It is used as an antacid *and* as a calcium supplement. Each Tums® contains about 200 mg of elemental calcium; however, Tums® does not supply the vitamin D that helps calcium absorption. *Remember: Your antacid (used for calcium supplementation) should not be taken with food.*

Calcium lactate is the best-absorbed supplement, but you need to take more calcium lactate than calcium carbonate because the percentage of elemental calcium that can be extracted is considerably lower than the amount released from calcium carbonate. The same is true of other calcium supplements, including calcium citrate, which is easier on the stomach, and calcium gluconate. Calcium must dissolve in your stomach to be absorbed. If your calcium tablet does not dissolve within thirty minutes, it will not be properly absorbed in your body.

Don't be confused by the labels on calcium products that may show the calcium compound and the amount of elemental calcium provided. You are interested in the latter number only. That's how much calcium you will actually receive.

Calcium Compound	Elemental Calcium Provided
Calcium Carbonate	40 percent
Calcium Citrate	21 percent
Calcium Lactate	13 percent
Calcium Gluconate	9 percent

The human body absorbs calcium most efficiently in amounts of 500 mg or less per dose. Absorption is always enhanced by taking your supplement with meals. You may hear that you should not take your calcium with meals if you eat a high-fiber diet, because fiber can reduce absorption. But all sources of fiber are not alike. Fiber found in fresh fruits, most vegetables, and grain products like oatmeal may indirectly help absorb calcium. The only foods that will interfere with the absorption of calcium are beans and foods high in oxalates, like spinach.

You can save money by purchasing tablets that deliver more than 500 mg of elemental calcium and breaking them in two. You can encourage absorption by drinking lots of water between meals.

Easy Science
You can find out how fast your calcium supplement will be absorbed using a mini-science experiment in your kitchen. Vinegar (which is acidic) mimics stomach acid. Put one tablet of your calcium supplement in 1/2 cup vinegar. Check it in one-half hour, and you'll find out how much calcium would be absorbed from your gastro-intestinal tract in the same amount of time. The absorbable part of the tablet will disintegrate, but it doesn't have to disappear. You never knew how easy it was to be a scientist, did you?

Many people are surprised to learn that calcium supplements can interact or bond with some foods and drugs. This binding process limits the availability of the calcium or the drug to your body. Spinach, beets, greens, chard, and rhubarb contain calcium-binding oxalates that decrease the absorption of calcium. Caffeine, iron, and unleavened grains also bind to calcium. On the days you add these foods to your diet, you need to take your calcium several hours before or after meals.

Calcium supplements and dairy products (the primary food source for calcium) also interact with many prescription drugs. These interactions can make the drugs less effective. If you are prescribed a drug that interacts with calcium, the bottle will be labeled with the warning "Do not take with dairy products." Some of the prescription drugs that interact unfavorably with calcium include

- Aluminum-containing antacids
- Antibiotics—tetracycline-based, quinolones, and gentiamicin
- Blood pressure medications—especially beta-blockers and calcium channel blockers
- Cholesterol-lowering drugs (some)
- Corticosteroids
- Digoxin
- Iron supplements (except calcium citrate)
- Seizure medications
- Thiazide and loop diuretics
- Thyroid medications

NOTE: For a complete list of interactions, use an Internet search engine and type in "calcium + drug interactions." Also see the Calcium Supplements and Drug Interactions chart in Appendix F.

Many people use calcium-based antacids as a calcium supplement. If you do, there are two things to remember:

1. Use the antacid at least one hour before or two hours after you eat, especially if you eat foods high in fiber or oxalates, which bind with the calcium and decrease absorption.
2. Be sure to fortify your diet with vitamin D (milk is a good source) or get at least fifteen minutes of sunlight on exposed skin.

Drug Interactions

Sophisticated pharmaceutical databases can predict drug and supplement interactions. When you use the same pharmacist for all your prescriptions, these databases will automatically generate a warning when drugs counteract or interact with one another. Telling your pharmacist when you add a supplement, herb, or over-the-counter product to your drug regimen assures that you will get the best and safest results from the medications you use. There are also on-line resources where patients can list their drugs and get this information.

Remember, calcium supplements can't cure osteoporosis. They support bone building and help prevent calcium removal from the bones. We agree with the recommended dietary intake of 1,200 to 1,500 mg/day. We prefer you get it from food, but taking 1,000 mg a day in a calcium supplement, in two divided doses of 500 mg each, is the best solution. Never take more than 2,500 mg a day. High doses increase the likelihood of developing kidney stones.

To benefit from calcium supplementation, choose a brand made by a reputable company. Don't skip your daily doses.

Increased awareness of the dangers of osteoporosis and the positive role calcium has in preventing the disease have brought all kinds of savvy marketers out of the woodwork. These entrepreneurs, eager to part you from your hard-earned dollars, describe their products with the words "purer" or "chelated" or "made from coral" or "patented in France." Often you are told they have secret formulas, are better absorbed, cure a wide range of diseases, and are "miracles."

You don't need these expensive products. The tried-and-true, inexpensive supplements are as good as they need to be. The money you can save is better put to use on a new pair of sturdy athletic shoes to support your exercise habit.

Sunshine and Vitamin D

Want to be sure you get the best absorption and use of calcium? Be sure you get enough vitamin D. Your body cannot absorb calcium from your intestine or make new bone without vitamin D. That doesn't mean you have to take vitamin D with calcium, but you do need to get it from some source.

You receive the vitamin D you need every day in two ways. The ultraviolet rays of the sun on your skin trigger the body's production of vitamin D. It takes about fifteen minutes of exposure every day for your skin to make the vitamin D your body needs. You also get vitamin D in your diet. The best source is fortified milk. (Yogurt, cottage cheese, and other milk products are not fortified with vitamin D.) It is also available in some fortified breakfast cereals. There is a lot of vitamin D in egg yolks and liver, but a lot of fat comes with it as well.

If you wear sunscreen (which protects you from skin cancer) or keep your skin covered anytime you are outside, or if an illness or injury keeps you housebound, your body will not get the ultraviolet rays necessary to make vitamin D. We also know the body's ability to make vitamin D declines with age. Vitamin D supplements then become a useful adjunct to your diet. Many multivitamin/mineral supplements have all the vitamin D you need, and many calcium supplements are packaged with vitamin D.

Like other fat-soluble vitamins (vitamin E, vitamin K, and vitamin A), vitamin D is measured in international units, or IU. We agree with dietary recommendations for 400 IU per day, unless you are at risk for osteoporosis or live where the sun does not appear much. Women whose cultures demand they cover their bodies also need the higher dosage. In that case, it is OK to double the dose to 800 IU per day.

Drink your milk and play outside, especially when it's sunny. After fifteen minutes in the sun, be sure to apply sunscreen. Take a general multivitamin/mineral product and a calcium and vitamin D supplement every day, and all your bases should be covered.

Other Vitamins and Minerals

Our bones contain many minerals in addition to calcium. Vitamin D, zinc, copper, manganese, boron, magnesium, and vitamin K all have roles in bone health. Calcium and other vitamins and minerals are also important in many other functions of the body in addition to bone health. As research about vitamins and minerals continues to evolve, it is certain we will learn about other micronutrients and the roles they play in the prevention and treatment of osteoporosis. For today, think diet first, then supplements. If you don't use dairy products, you can take care of your calcium needs with a general multivitamin/mineral tablet and calcium supplement. If you want to take a stress vitamin (B vitamins) and/or an antioxidant (vitamin C, vitamin E, or zinc), it won't hurt you. If you break the pharmacist Ronda's "rule of five," (taking more than five products each day), you are in overkill and should check with your pharmacist about possible interactions.

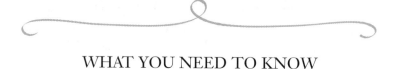

WHAT YOU NEED TO KNOW

Supplements can play a vital role in ensuring that you get nutrients missing in your diet because of chronic illness, dieting, stress, or poor eating habits. Supplements can also pump up the vitamin and mineral content of a decent diet, especially if taken with food in a form that assures they will be well absorbed.

Calcium, the most abundant mineral in the body, cannot cure osteoporosis; however, a calcium-rich diet and calcium supplements can assure bone calcium is not compromised when the body is challenged by other needs for calcium. Your body cannot absorb more than 500 mg of calcium at a time, so if you rely on a supplement to get calcium, take it at least twice a day. Check supplement bottles for the amount of elemental calcium the supplement truly delivers.

Vitamin D plays an important role in the absorption of calcium. Fifteen minutes of exposure to the sun every day can trigger your body to produce

the vitamin D you need. Supplementation of vitamin D in the form of fortified foods or the small amount available in a multivitamin/mineral tablet
can provide useful insurance, especially for people who live in gray winter
climates, use sunscreen, keep their skin covered, or are bedridden. Many
calcium supplements come with vitamin D added.

Exercise:
One More Time for Good Measure

We believe it is essential to understand the principles underlying good advice. For exercise, this includes basic knowledge about how your body works. Armed with this information, you can make an informed decision about which exercise strategy is best for your overall good health, including the strength and density of your bones. When your motivation lags or someone tempts you with a quick exercise fix with a magic machine, you can rely on this knowledge to retain self-mastery of your fitness strategy.

A Brief Review

Each fall when trees lose their leaves, homeowners face the awesome task of raking them up and hauling them away. If they tackle the job in one weekend, repetitive raking can produce painful blisters that eventually heal, leaving no telltale signs of the effort. But suppose the leaves on the tree fell all year long and our homeowner faced a little bit of leaf raking every day. Instead of blisters you would see calluses.

As you learned in chapter 10, daily aerobic exercise can strengthen bones. Choose your exercise wisely and the repetitive "strike force" or impact of your foot (bearing the weight of your body on a hard surface) reminds your bones to get thicker and harder so they will be less prone to injury when stressed. It's this impact that is important. Nonimpact exercise on bicycles or elliptical exercise machines or in water will make you fit; you will even gain some increase in bone density from the effort required to push a pedal or pull your arm through water. But these activities don't bear your weight, so they won't harden bone as effectively as weight-bearing walking, jogging, stair climbing, step aerobics, and dancing. Don't misquote us: we think non–weight-bearing exercises are great for fitness, but we don't think they are the best choice for bones.

Magnitude of Force + Frequency of Application

creates

Mechanical Stress

and

Electrical Energy

that

Stimulates the Bone

and

Increases the Calcium Content of Bone

resulting in

Bone Hypertrophy (thicker bones)

In chapter 10 you also learned that bone strength is directly proportionate to the strength of the attached muscles. If you put a rubber band on the end of a stick and pull, you must stabilize the stick to keep it from bending or snapping. If you have a thick stick, you can be less concerned about breakage. The beauty of the relationship between muscle and bone is that when muscles get stronger, bones do, too. That's why, in addition to high- or low-impact aerobic exercise, doctors are now encouraging women to add anaerobic upper- and lower-body strength training to their fitness routines.

Last, but not least, activities that improve balance, coordination, and flexibility are important if you want to avoid falls. Yoga, tai chi, Pilates, and the martial arts also improve core muscle strength in the abdominal and pelvic region. This contributes to better posture, a feeling of stability when standing or walking, and ease in completing daily chores.

Fueling Your Engine

Like a car, your muscles require fuel to work. With a car, you can choose the octane of the gas you use, but the fuel is *always* gas. Your muscles have a choice of two fuels—fat in the form of fatty acids, the primary fuel in aerobic exercise, or sugar in the form of glucose, the primary fuel in anaerobic exercise. You get the fat from the meat, milk, and whole grains you eat as well as from any fat you add to foods. You get the sugar from fruits, vegetables, whole grains, and any sugar you add to foods. Both fuels are used, but the preference of one over the other depends on the intensity of your effort. Your diet also includes protein provided by meat, milk, soy, eggs, nuts, and beans; however, muscles don't like to use protein for the work they do. They use the protein after the workout, when they respond to your effort by strengthening muscles.

Macronutrient/fuel	Foods
Carbohydrates	Fruits, vegetables, whole grains, and added sugars
Fat	Meat, whole milk and whole-milk products, added fats including butter, margarine, and salad dressings
Protein	Meat, poultry, fish, milk and milk products, and eggs

Regardless of your food choice—carbohydrate, fat, or protein—the energy in food is measured in calories. Some of that caloric energy is used right away. Any extra is stored in your body until you need it. A limited amount of sugar energy (glucose) is stored in the liver. Fat, on the other hand, has no limits on the amount that can be stored.

Some of us have too much stored energy. The only advantage to this abundant storage, or being overweight, is that overweight people have stronger bones to support that extra weight. If you are overweight, you may be happy to hear this news. Before you get too excited, remember that the many health consequences of being overweight far outweigh this single advantage.

Bone-building Exercise Burns Calories

Most women we meet are eager to maintain a healthy weight. They ask why they begin to gain weight as they approach menopause. After menopause they wonder why the amount and location of that weight seems to shift upward. There is no easy answer to these questions because our ability to gain or lose weight easily is based on complex factors. Like osteoporosis, weight gain doesn't happen overnight. If you aren't exercising regularly, your metabolism slows down as you age and your muscle also yields to that "use it or lose it" mantra. If you have less muscle, your body uses fewer calories. In time that can add up to additional stored fat. Health specialists also know that estrogen is made from and stored in body fat. If our estrogen levels are decreasing, perhaps our body is striving to keep estrogen levels high by holding on to extra fat.

Despite the complex issues involved, weight management, for most of us, is nothing more than balancing calories in and calories out. A deprivation model that restricts calories, food groups, and the nutrients your body needs can be hazardous to your bones and other health systems. Instead, turn your attention to using stored fuel with your weight-bearing aerobic and anaerobic exercise program. You do this by customizing *your* program by varying it in three ways. There's an acronym that makes this easy to understand. It's FIT:

F = frequency, or how often you exercise
I = intensity, or how hard you exercise
T = time, or how long you exercise

You have several choices:

1. Exercise frequently, but not hard or for very long
2. Exercise with intensity so you don't have to exercise as often or as long
3. Exercise for a long time so you don't have to exercise as often or as hard

Here's how it works. If you exercise often, hard, and for long periods of time, you are more prone to injury. If you exercise rarely, at a low intensity, and for short periods of time, it will be a long time before you see results. As in most activities, moderation is the best course of action.

Some exercise specialists add a second T (for technique) to FIT to describe the kind of exercise you choose. For treating osteoporosis, this is the aerobic and anaerobic weight-bearing exercise so important to bones.

If you exercise at this FREQUENCY	and your INTENSITY is	the suggested amount of TIME of the exercise session should be	for this suggested TECHNIQUE
2–3 times a day	low to moderate	10–15 minutes	walk, low-impact aerobics, tennis, exercise machine
daily	moderate to hard	30–40 minutes	jog/run, step aerobics, climbing stairs
daily	low to moderate	60–90 minutes	walk

One More Time

Suppose that you stood up and, holding on to a chair, bent your knee and lifted your leg and then lowered it, repeatedly. After a while the muscle doing that work, called a hip flexor, might get tired, but chances are you wouldn't get warm from your effort. You might argue that the exercise meets aerobic guidelines for using big muscles in the lower body and that it meets weight-bearing standards because you are on your feet. But since the effort is so localized, other body systems don't work very hard. Suppose, instead, that you sat in a chair, then stood up and sat down ten or twenty times. Chances are you would start to get breathless and warm because so many muscles are being used.

Standing up and sitting down is a good aerobic exercise because the big muscles of the lower body are being used, but, once again, to help bones, the goal is *impact*. If you marched in place twenty times each time you stood up, you would be doing the bones and muscles of your lower body a big favor. Regardless of what aerobic exercise you choose, keep thinking as you move, "Grow, osteoblasts, grow."

The anaerobic workout you do with weights or resistance bands has another advantage in addition to strengthening bones. It boosts your metabolism. A higher metabolism burns more calories per minute whether you are sitting around or working out. In other words, the more muscle you have, the more calories you burn per minute. You can boost your metabolism the way athletes do. Add sprints to your aerobic program. You do this by exercising at the aerobic pace that makes you slightly breathless (but not out of breath), then taking your effort up a notch until you are breathless, which signals the body to switch from fat-burning aerobic metabolism to glucose-burning anaerobic metabolism. Slow down until you catch your breath; then exert yourself again. This "interval training" helps you get fit fast and burns extra calories after the workout. It also will help you manage your weight.

Now that you understand the principles behind a bone-building workout, use the following guidelines to customize your personal program.

1. Find an exercise that you enjoy. Better yet, to fulfill a goal for cross-training, find several activities that give you pleasure. That's the only way to assure you will keep going back for more.

2. Start slowly. This prevents injuries. You may be enthusiastic and want to conquer this disease as soon as possible, but Rome wasn't built in a day. Neither is a fit, strong body. Your effort should progress until you are moving longer, more often, and with sufficient intensity to help those bones.

A graduated walking program is a good place for beginners to start. Walk alone or walk with friends. Use the walking program in Appendix G to assure you get the best from your efforts to support stronger bones without a risk of injury.

3. Be patient. Adults are funny. They spend a lot of time teaching children patience, then neglect the lesson themselves. Instead of attempting to whip yourself into shape in a few weeks, progress slowly. If you want to avoid sore muscles, you are likely to say, "Hmmm . . . that wasn't so bad; maybe tomorrow I'll go a little farther or faster or longer."

4. Exercise often. The benefits of exercise are achieved when you consistently pursue your goal. Essentially, you remind your muscles, "This activity is going to happen on a regular basis." They respond by getting fitter. If you are just getting started, exercise for short periods of time, several times a day, at least five days a week. Once you get fit you can sustain your fitness level by being active three times a week, but bone-building results require frequency of effort. When you set a plan, remember there is no *right* time to exercise. Some experts encourage morning exercise, which keeps metabolism high all day. Others encourage exercise late in the day to burn more calories while you sleep. Instead of worrying about which choice will give you the best results, exercise at the time of day that assures you will stick with your program. If you build exercise into your day by walking and climbing instead of driving, parking farther from destinations, and doing the physical work of house and garden maintenance instead of relying on machines or other people, you may find you don't have to add "workout time" to your daily schedule.

Fitness experts remind us that it takes 6,000 steps a day to gain health benefits and at least 10,000 steps a day to get fit and lose weight. Most people, especially those who lead a sedentary lifestyle, take less than 1,500 steps a day. If you want to outwit osteoporosis, get a pedometer to make sure you meet the 10,000-step-a-day bone-building guidelines.

5. Break a rule. When it comes to intensity, ignore the formula that takes your age into consideration. Your current fitness level, not your age, should determine your exercise pace. You should be slightly breathless during aerobic fitness and have intervals of breathlessness during anaerobic fitness. When strength training, stop just short of "the burn." Pay attention to how you feel as you exercise. On a good day, when your routine is comfortable, push yourself a little harder. If you don't feel up to par another day, take it easy, but *keep doing something*.

Even after many years of daily workouts, there are still days when your authors do not want to exercise. We operate with the following philosophy. *The first day we don't exercise is the first day of poor habit building we will regret later*. Now we know that after we get our blood pumping and return home, we are *always* glad we put in the effort.

6. Do ANYTHING to help yourself stick with your program. Set short- and long-term goals that motivate rather than discourage you. Some people like the structure of a planned program, and record keeping helps them measure their progress. Other people like to go with the flow and decide on a daily basis what they are going to do and when they will do it. Some people like group exercise and others prefer exercising alone. The options are as varied as people are.

WHAT YOU NEED TO KNOW

A focus on the underlying principles of aerobic and anaerobic metabolism can be a motivating factor when you design an exercise program to prevent (and treat) osteoporosis. If you use aerobic *and* anaerobic fitness principles you will get fit fast, increase your metabolism, *and* build strong bones. The acronym FITT (frequency, intensity, time, and technique) is a good way to design a program. If you find an exercise you enjoy, start slowly, are patient, exercise consistently, pace yourself accordingly, and focus on goals, you can be assured you are well on your way to outwitting osteoporosis.

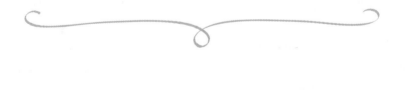

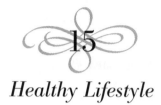

Healthy Lifestyle

We've covered all the dietary and lifestyle issues that are important for the prevention of osteoporosis except for two: smoking and stress reduction.

Smoking—Again

Not long ago, smoking was cool. There were ashtrays on restaurant tables and circular sand-filled bins in front of elevator doors in department stores. Back then you could even smoke in an airplane. Then a shift began. We remember the early days of that shift. Friends and relatives with the cigarette habit criticized Ronda for posting and enforcing a "no smoking" sign in her home. Beverly remembers visits by her mother, who stood in front of the Whipple home, cigarette in hand, complaining to every passing neighbor about her "mean daughter" who wouldn't let her smoke in the house.

My, how times have changed! Tobacco companies now admit they added addictive nicotine to cigarettes. Many states require that public places must be smoke-free. Although there are still mini-ashtrays on the arms of airplane seats and in their lavatories, if you light up, you will set off alarms and be evicted at the next stop. People who smoke at work must do it outside of the building. Smoke one pack of cigarettes a day for twenty years and it's almost certain you will get lung cancer. Smoking kills.

In chapter 5 you learned that smoking is a serious risk factor for osteoporosis. Nicotine increases estrogen breakdown and decreases the population of osteoblasts. If you smoke, you are more likely to go through menopause earlier, depriving your body of a few additional years of bone-strengthening estrogen protection.

If you smoke, stop. We agree it's easier said than done, but there are excellent programs and products to support withdrawal. If you don't smoke, don't start. It isn't cool. It's deadly. (See the Resources section for support to help you stop smoking.)

Stress Reduction

Your emotional outlook and attitude can affect how you deal with the lifestyle changes that prevent or treat osteoporosis. The key is taking care of yourself.

Set aside time each day (even if it is just a few minutes) for relaxation. Reaffirm your intent for a healthy lifestyle. Attempt to release negative feelings. Mentally, give your stress away or symbolically put it into something you can safely destroy. The emerging research about the physiological and psychological benefits gained by brief breaks, reflective time, mental exercise, and recreation can't be denied.

Consider the use of affirmations to support new bone-building habits. At first, the use of this behavior-changing tool may feel uncomfortable. "How can I affirm what isn't true?" "This feels awkward," or "I think this is stupid" are just a few of the comments we hear when we make this suggestion.

Use the following guidelines to get started:

- Begin your affirmation with the word "I." This is a strong statement of your personal power.

- Always affirm in the present. Instead of saying "My bones are getting stronger," say, "My bones are stronger."
- Omit the word "should" from affirmations. Instead of "I should," say, "I do."
- Avoid using the words "no," "non," "not," and "never." "I no longer fall down," or "I never fall," are powerful reminders you have changed, but they are negative. More positive choices are "I am poised and confident and have steady feet" or "I have excellent balance."
- Avoid using the words "hope," wish," and "try." They are vague and suggest the possibility of failure. Have you ever "tried" to pick up your car keys? No—you just reach out and pick them up! It is much easier and it takes less energy to do things than to "try to" or "want to" or "need to" do them. Instead of "I am trying to exercise every day," or "I want to exercise every day," affirm, "I exercise daily."
- Don't slip into self-abusive speaking patterns. Whenever you catch yourself using this kind of language, add the phrase "up until now." It reverses the self-defeating message about to be stored in your brain. "I always forget to take my calcium supplement" becomes "I always forget to take my calcium supplement, up until now."

After you create your affirmation, repeat it to yourself several times. If it feels somewhat comfortable, you have chosen well. Most people need to adjust the wording of their affirmation until it seems "right."

Here are some affirmations that have worked for many women:

- "I care about myself and my body."
- "Every day I do what is necessary to be healthy."

- "I exercise, eat smart, and take my calcium to prevent osteoporosis."
- "I stand straight and tall. I have no fractures."

WHAT YOU NEED TO KNOW

A healthy lifestyle is a smoke-free lifestyle. It also includes strategies to manage stress, a positive attitude, and a consistent effort to affirm and practice habits that say "I care about myself."

Section V

Osteoporosis–
Not Just a Woman's Disease

Osteoporosis in Men

Dave, age 52, a physically active man, recently went to his doctor for a checkup. Like most men his age, his concerns were his blood pressure, his cholesterol reading, and the health of his colon and prostate. But he also told his doctor, "I know I carry my stress in my upper back, neck, and shoulders, but the pain I've had there lately is pretty intense." The doctor referred him for X rays. When the results came back, Dave was stunned to learn he had compression fractures in his upper back. His doctor told him, "You have osteoporosis."

"That's impossible," Dave said. "I run three or four miles every day."

Running is a very good fitness routine. It can prevent the heart, colon, and prostate diseases that concerned Dave. It can also strengthen the hips and lower spine, but it doesn't do much to strengthen the upper back.

Like most people we meet, Dave thought osteoporosis was a woman's disease. He'd seen a few stooped older men but had attributed their stature to aging. He had never realized that a man his age had to worry about his bones.

It is true that osteoporosis is diagnosed less often in men than in women, but the statistics for its occurrence are not something to overlook.

- According to the National Osteoporosis Foundation, two million American men have osteoporosis. An additional twelve million are at risk for the disease. That number is expected to swell to more than twenty million by 2020.

- Worldwide, the International Osteoporosis Foundation reports that the lifetime risk for low-trauma, osteoporotic fractures in men is 25 percent. This translates to one in four men over age fifty having an osteoporosis-related fracture in their lifetime.
- Worldwide, the risk for hip fractures in men is higher than that of prostate cancer.
- Men, whose osteoporosis and subsequent hip fractures tend to occur at an older age when they may be less active and already sick, are more likely than women to die after a hip fracture.
- More than 50 percent of men with hip fractures go from the hospital to a nursing home. Of those who survive the first year, 79 percent never return home.
- Men who smoke have a greater risk for osteoporosis.
- Alcoholics have a much higher incidence of osteoporosis than non-drinkers.

Until recently, most health research, including that for heart disease, stroke, and cancer, was conducted on men and the results were extrapolated to women. In 1993 legislation changed that. Researchers quickly realized that it would be easy to secure funding for diseases seen more often in women—especially postmenopausal women whose health seemed to deteriorate as their estrogen levels dropped dramatically. Osteoporosis came to attention because women who were living longer were often becoming debilitated or dying after a hip fracture. The disease wasn't seen so often in men. When it was, the men tended to be older and often already sick with something else. Many men are now paying the price for this reverse prejudice.

Men have larger and stronger skeletons than women, so they have a slight edge when it comes to the bone loss that accompanies aging. In fact, most men don't get fragile bones or the osteoporosis diagnosis until much later in life than women. That diagnosis usually occurs when, like Dave, they go to a doctor for back pain or have an unexpected fracture and the doctor, who suspects osteoporosis, does a bone scan that reveals the disease.

Men also don't have the abrupt drop in estrogen production that women experience at menopause, but they do have estrogen and that estrogen level does decline with age. The primary sexual hormone in men is testosterone. Testosterone probably has positive effects on bones. We know it gives men bigger muscles, which indirectly results in a higher bone density. Additionally, some of that testosterone gets converted to estrogen, which prevents the excessive osteoclast activity that resorbs bone. When a man's testosterone or estrogen level drops (or if he has low hormone levels to start with), he will experience bone loss. If he isn't physically active, he will lose bone. If he also smokes, uses alcohol excessively, doesn't eat calcium-rich foods, or has a family history for osteoporosis, he may lose much more. The ethnic risk for osteoporosis in men is similar to that of women. Non-Hispanic, Caucasian, and Asian men have the greatest risk for osteoporosis, but men of all ethnic groups can get osteoporosis.

> Too few men get dual-energy X ray absorptiometry measurements. Men who experience decreased sexual function due to low testosterone levels should have a DEXA scan to measure bone density.

Other situations that should prompt a bone density measurement for a man include:

1. A low-trauma fracture (for instance, due to a fall from standing height or less)
2. Taking a medication known to cause bone loss
3. Having a medical illness that can affect the strength of the skeleton

As Dave learned more about osteoporosis, he wondered if early use of a corticosteroid to treat his asthma was the predisposing factor to his disease. "It's possible," his doctor told him. "Most doctors will admit that they neglect to pay attention to the fact that long-term treatment with steroids or other drugs could compromise bone health. Now we know that—in addition to low production of hormones and aging—treatment for intestinal disorders, cancer, or diseases that require the use of corticosteroids is also a hallmark of the medical history of men with osteoporosis."

In addition to a DEXA scan to measure bone density, Dave received a prescription to treat his fracture pain, and was sent to a physical therapist who agreed to help him design an upper-body weight-training program once his pain diminished. Dave began taking a calcium and vitamin D supplement twice a day. He also joined one of the drug trials that is studying the use of parathyroid hormone (PHT) to treat osteoporosis. His prognosis is good.

Treatment

Men have an additional disadvantage when it comes to treatment for their disease: They don't have the range of treatment choices afforded to women.

Estrogen isn't an option for men. Alendronate (Fosamax®) has been approved, and studies are under way to see if risedronate (Actonel®) should be added to the list of treatment options for men. Both are already approved to treat glucocorticoid-induced osteoporosis in men (and in women). PTH (Forteo® by Eli Lilly & Co.) has been approved to increase bone mass in men with primary or hypogonadal osteoporosis who are at high risk for a fracture. Men who have had bone density assessments before and after treatment with testosterone get the good news that the drug helps their bones. Other drugs for women, such as sodium fluoride, vitamin D metabolites, other bisphosphonates, and SERMs, are still under investigation for use by men.

There is also an explosion of support groups for men—especially on the Internet. See the Resources section for details.

A Coincidence

While we were writing this book, a friend put Ronda in touch with Dr. Eric Orwoll, a physician and osteoporosis researcher at Oregon Health & Science University. Serendipity prevailed. It turned out that Dr. Orwoll was heading a National Institutes of Health (NIH) study on men and osteoporosis. Six thousand men have been recruited and will be followed for a number of years. It's one of the largest studies on men and osteoporosis to date.

Ronda asked Dr. Orwoll, "What are the most important things we should mention in our book?" He responded, "The research on new treatments (like PTH), the emerging statistics about incidence of osteoporosis in men, and the need to encourage men and their physicians to take advantage of DEXA measurements to detect the disease in men."

Prevention

Because men have bigger bones and lose bone mass at a slower rate than women, they have much more time to prevent the disease. If they haven't adopted an osteoporosis-savvy lifestyle, it's not too late to start. Exercise is mandatory. The aerobic/anaerobic/flexibility/coordination/balance programs you read about in chapter 14 apply here. Men also need a balanced, varied, low-in-fat, low-in-sugar, and high-in-fiber diet. They need adequate calcium in their diet but not so much that they increase their risk for prostate cancer. The typical guideline is 1,200 to 1,500 mg per day. If they don't get at least fifteen minutes of sun a day, they need a vitamin D supplement to support calcium absorption. Smoking is prohibited, and alcohol consumption should be limited to two drinks a day. Men (and women) who use antacids should avoid products that contain aluminum or magnesium.

DEXA scans can detect osteoporosis before a fracture occurs. They are recommended for men who have low testosterone levels, a fracture, curvature of the spine, loss of height, or back pain, or if they have one of the medical conditions or have taken any of the medications that affect bone mass.

WHAT YOU NEED TO KNOW

Men of all ages and the women who love them need to pay attention to Dave's story. Men have considerable risk for osteoporosis, but because their bones and muscles are larger to start with and because they lose bone more slowly than women, they have a better opportunity than women to prevent this disease. If they experience a fracture or have a medical condition that requires medications that predispose them to osteoporosis (especially corticosteroids), they should have a DEXA scan. If diagnosed with osteopenia or osteoporosis, their treatment options are similar to those of women.

Happily, there is extensive research being conducted to learn more about how to prevent and treat "the silent thief" in men *and* women. None of us want to be blindsided by something that can be as devastating as osteoporosis. Taking a proactive approach to total health, including maintaining bone health, can change the course of your health history.

Section VI

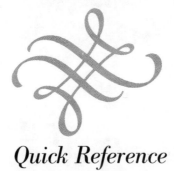

Quick Reference

Questions and Answers

We always smile when someone approaches us after a lecture and says, "I have a quick question." Quick questions rarely require quick answers. Since many are repeated often, we've included some of them here in the hopes that one will apply to your specific problem.

I'm forty-five years old. When do I need to start worrying about the health of my bones?

Worrying about your bone health serves no useful purpose. Instead, we encourage a proactive lifestyle approach that begins as soon as a woman learns how important strong bones are to her lifelong health. Since the habits forged early in life set the stage for adult health, we encourage mothers who ask their children, "Did you brush your teeth?" and "Did you wash your hands?" to add, "Did you do something for your bones today?"

Why is osteoporosis called "the silent thief"?

Bones begin their development in utero and, under normal circumstances, keep developing rapidly after birth until we are about thirty years old. After that, bone mass stabilizes for a few years until the activity of osteoblast cells that increase bone density declines and the activity of osteoclast cells that decrease bone density persists. That results in a bone loss of about 1 percent a year until perimenopause, when declining levels of estrogen further accelerate bone loss. Bone loss, for many women, is heightened again in the first few years after menopause. Since a woman can't see her skeleton, there is no way of knowing if she has experienced bone loss—unless she has a bone density assessment. If bone loss has occurred, we can say she's been robbed by a silent thief.

I just had a DEXA scan, with normal results. Am I safe?

A DEXA scan measures your bone density accurately on the day you have the assessment. Your bone status can begin to change at any time. We recommend a premenopausal baseline DEXA scan to set a benchmark, to which any future assessments can be compared. If your second assessment is also normal, you can wait up to five years for your next assessment. When there is a significant change in bone density, we recommend the scan be repeated within two years.

If my mother and grandmother both had dowager's humps at age seventy-five, am I genetically doomed to be stooped over, too?

Absolutely not. The weak upper back and dowager's hump that is diagnostic for osteoporosis is preventable. If you haven't started weight-bearing exercises yet, start today. Add calcium-rich foods to your diet and use a calcium and vitamin D supplement daily. Get a bone scan to get a baseline score to which future assessments can be compared. If you are postmenopausal, ask your doctor if you are a candidate for osteoporosis prevention therapy.

Is it true that when I get old I will be frail and weak and there is nothing I can do about it?

No. You have almost everything to do with the quality of your life in the future. Disease is a process. If you keep active and healthy, you can avoid the weakness that has, in the past, been a hallmark of old age. We cheer the active aging who disagree with folks who say, "You're too old to do that."

Is it true that once I have lost bone, it is gone forever?

No. When bone loss is detected early enough, proper medication, supplements, and changes in lifestyle can encourage the growth of new bone.

My daughter rolls her eyes and sighs when I say, "I got osteoporosis at age eighty." What is her point?

Many people don't realize that most diseases take a long time to progress sufficiently to produce symptoms. This is especially true of osteoporosis, which rages silently before a DEXA scan or a fracture precipitates the diagnosis. Perhaps your daughter remembers your lengthy years of poor lifestyle habits that may have triggered your disease. That is why it is so important, in our early years, to live the kind of life that assures we are doing the best we can to prepare ourselves for a life of active aging.

How can I help my children and grandchildren prevent osteoporosis?

Teach your children and grandchildren that most of the diseases of aging, including osteoporosis, don't happen overnight. Remind them that most diseases progress silently until there is a crisis that reveals the results of poor lifestyle choices at an earlier age. This is particularly true with osteoporosis.

Encourage them to drink milk instead of juice or soda pop, eat a healthy diet, and avoid dieting, smoking, and excessive use of alcohol. Provide smart guidance about the supplements they can use to synergize the good lifestyle habits that can build and maintain bone and prevent osteoporosis (and other diseases of aging). And, as you teach, practice what you preach.

Won't I gain weight on a calcium-rich diet?

Smart eating includes the use of high-in-calcium dairy products that are also low in fat and sugar. You actually get more calcium in a serving of nonfat milk (80 calories) than you do in a serving of whole milk (156 calories). The same is true for other skim and low-fat milk-based products, including cheese, yogurt, and low-fat frozen desserts, so you and your family can enjoy them without worrying about gaining weight. Of course, you must exercise and be sure that you don't eat more calories than you burn. That's what weight management is about—balancing the intake and output of calories.

How do I know which drug is right for me?

You and your health-care provider are partners in determining which medication is right for you. This is based on your health history, your risk factors, and the results of your DEXA scan.

How much calcium do my children and I need?

The National Institutes of Health's Developmental Conference on Optimal Calcium Intake makes the following recommendations:

Ages 1–3:   500 mg/day
Ages 4–8:   800 mg/day

Ages 9–18:   1,300 mg/day

Age 19–50:   Prior to menopause: 1,000 mg/day

                        Premature menopause: 1,500 mg/day

Age 50–65:   After menopause with estrogen therapy:

                        1,000 to 1,200 mg/day

                        After menopause without estrogen therapy:

                        1,500 mg/day

Over Age 65:   1,500 mg/day

How much calcium does my infant need?

Infants from birth to six months need 210 mg of calcium per day, and infants from six months to one year need 270 mg per day.

Do I need more calcium when I am pregnant or breast-feeding?

Pregnant and lactating women will need to add 400 mg per day to the above doses.

Is it possible to take too much calcium?

Most experts are not worried about the risk of excessive intake, but also recommend that you don't routinely exceed 2,500 mg per day. For the best absorption, space your calcium intake throughout the day.

I can't exercise. What can I do to help prevent osteoporosis?

Sorry. We don't buy the "can't exercise" excuse. Unless you can't move, there is something you can do. Work with a sports-medicine physician or physical therapist to find a way to overcome your barriers. This is especially important for women who have weak muscles.

My mother was diagnosed with osteoporosis. She's on medication and sees a physical therapist. Do you have any other suggestions to support her care?

Since falls are so dangerous for people who have osteoporosis, here are some tips that can make your mother's living environment safer:

- Be sure all carpets, especially area rugs, have skid-proof backings.
- If a floor is waxed, it is slippery. Give up the shine.
- Install grab bars in the bathroom to make sitting down, standing up, and moving in and out of a tub or shower safer.
- Spend time with your mother so you can identify which items she uses frequently. Then put them within easy reach. This includes pens, pencils, notepads, soap and toilet paper in the bathroom, and food in the refrigerator.
- If your mother is unsteady, buy her a cane or walker to support her confidence to keep moving.

I have three small children. I am almost always carrying one of them. Is that enough weight-bearing exercise?

Carrying children is good weight-bearing exercise, but it is not enough to prevent osteoporosis because you are doing only one kind of lifting. To prevent osteoporosis you need to strengthen your upper-body muscles in several ways. The books listed in the Resources section will give you all the information you need.

Also be sure you understand that "weight bearing" describes two different kinds of exercise. In addition to the strength training suggested above, it is important to move your feet.

Experts often argue about which is best for bones. Instead of choosing one, do both. Strength (or resistance) train *and* get into a physical activity program that requires your foot to strike a hard surface. Walking, jogging, stepping, kick boxing, and dancing are just a few of the options that work well when you want to build and maintain bone. (See Ronda's Smart Walking program on page 187.)

Appendices

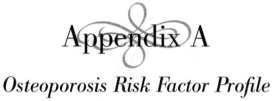

Appendix A

Osteoporosis Risk Factor Profile

To help determine your risk of osteoporosis, circle the number in each category next to the statement that is most true for you. Add up the points when you have finished the entire profile.

Genetic Factors

Age:

Under 35	1
35–50	3
51–65	7
Over 65	12

Heritage:

African American	1
Asian	2
Mediterranean or Middle Eastern	3
Caucasian	5

Complexion:

Dark	1
Ruddy/Olive	2
Fair/Pale	3

Family History:

No known bone problems in family	1
Relative over age 60 with bone disease	3
Parent with bone disease	4
Relative under age 60 with bone disease	5

Wrist Size:

Over 6.5″	1
6–6.5″	2
5–6″	3
Under 5″	4

Height:

Over 5′8″	1
5′5″–5′8″	2
5′2″–5′5″	3
Under 5′2″	4

Body Type:

Mesomorphic (high muscle, low fat)	1
Endomorphic (high fat, low muscle)	6
Ectomorphic (low fat, low muscle)	6

Onset of Menopause:

After age 50	1
Age 46–50	3
Age 45 or under*	5
Surgical menopause age 45 or under*	7

*Deduct 5 points if estrogen therapy started within one year after surgery or early menopause. Deduct 3 points if estrogen therapy started more than three years after surgery or early menopause.

My Genetic Score   _____

Lifestyle Factors

Exercise (total body):

Four or more times a week	0
One to three times a week	3
At least 3 times a month	6
Avoid physical activity	12

Calcium Intake:

Four or more servings of low-fat dairy products a day	0
More than 2 servings a day	3
Two or fewer servings a day	6
Avoid dairy products	12

Protein Intake:

Avoid red meat	0
Eat only seafood and white meat poultry	1
Eat meat 3 times a week or less	3
Eat meat 4 times a week or more	6

Caffeine Consumption:

Avoid caffeine and tannin beverages	0
Drink decaffeinated drinks and/or tea only	2
Drink 3 cups or less of coffee/tea daily	3
Drink 4 cups or more coffee daily	6

Alcohol Consumption:

    Less than 2 beers, 8 oz. wine, or 3 oz. of spirits per week   0

    Two to four beers, 8–16 oz. wine, or 3–6 oz. spirits per week 2

    Up to 2 beers, 8 oz. wine, or 3 oz. spirits per day   4

    More than 2 beers, 16 oz. wine, or 6 oz. spirits per day   8

Tobacco Use:

    Nonsmoker   0

    Less than 14 cigarettes per week   2

    Less than 10 cigarettes per day   5

    Ten cigarettes or more per day   8

My Lifestyle Score   _____

+

My Genetic Score   _____

=

My Total Score   _____

What your score means:

  8–25 points: Your risk factor is well below average.

  26–48 points: Your risk factor is average.

  49–82 points: You are at moderate risk for developing osteoporosis.

  83–100 points: You are at a considerable risk for developing osteoporosis.

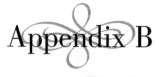

Appendix B

Osteoporosis Risk Factors

Abnormal absence of menstrual periods

Advanced age

Anorexia nervosa or bulimia

Caucasian or Asian race (although African Americans and Hispanic
Americans are also at risk)

Chronic use of steroids, excessive thyroid hormone, and certain
anticonvulsants

Early menopause (before age forty-five)

Excessive use of alcohol

Excessive use of caffeine

Family history of osteoporosis

Menopause

No pregnancies

Sedentary lifestyle

Thin or small frame

Use of tobacco

Insufficient milk, especially between ages of one through sixteen

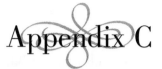

Appendix C

What to Do for Your Bones as You Age

(Note: Ranges in calcium recommendation reflect differences in sources of recommendations.)

Up to Ten Years Old

Bone Activity

Bones are developing, growing rapidly; bone-building osteoblasts are more active than bone-draining osteoclasts; soft plates in skull harden and expand

Diet

Whole milk in the first two years of life, then 2 percent or nonfat milk and milk products; minimize juice and soda as beverages of choice; encourage diet of whole grains, fruits, and vegetables; avoid foods that have more calories than nutrients

Calcium

Infant to 6 months: 210 mg; 6 months to 1 year: 270 mg; 1–3 years: 500 mg; 4–8 years: 800 mg; 9–10 years: 1,300 mg

In Your Teens

Bone Activity
Bones are continuing to grow, with focus of cell activity on bone length; osteoblast activity exceeds osteoclast activity

Diet
No dieting—any weight management is a function of exercise and a focus on healthy whole foods, such as whole grains, fresh fruits and vegetables, chicken, fish, and lean meats; minimize foods with added fat or sugar

Calcium
11–18: 1,300 mg; 19–20: 1,000 mg

Lifestyle
Don't succumb to peer pressure to smoke or use alcoholic beverages; participation in athletic activities mandatory

In Your Twenties

Bone Activity

Growth is finished; osteoblast activity is focused on increasing bone density; osteoclast activity surpasses osteoclast activity; surgical- or drug-induced menopause can precipitate drop in bone-stabilizing estrogen levels

Diet

Focus on healthy whole foods, such as whole grains, fresh fruits and egetables, chicken, fish, and lean meats; minimize foods with added fat or sugar

Calcium

Add a supplement to ensure 1,000 mg/day calcium intake. If supplementing with more than 500 mg calcium, the pills should be in divided doses

Lifestyle

Daily weight-bearing exercise mandatory; be aware of potential for mandatory drug regimen to affect bones

In Your Thirties

Bone Activity
Bone mass stabilizes; activity of osteoblast cells decreases; bone density can be maintained or decreased based on diet, exercise, or medication; surgical- or drug-induced menopause can precipitate drop in bone-stabilizing estrogen levels

Diet
Focus on healthy whole foods, such as whole grains, fresh fruits and vegetables, chicken, fish, and lean meats; minimize foods with added fat or sugar

Calcium
1,000 mg

Lifestyle
If menopause induced by presurgical or drug treatment, DEXA scan recommended to get baseline bone density measurements; be sure exercise program includes strength or resistance training

In Your Forties

Bone Activity

Bone density subject to osteoclast activity outpaces osteoblast activity; estrogen levels drop; bone density can be maintained or decreased based on diet, exercise, or medication; surgical- or drug-induced menopause can precipitate drop in bone-stabilizing estrogen levels

Diet

Focus on healthy whole foods, such as whole grains, fresh fruits and vegetables, chicken, fish, and lean meats; minimize foods with added fat or sugar

Calcium

1,000–1,200 mg

Lifestyle

DEXA scan to ensure a knowledge of baseline bone density; begin proactive discussion with doctor about postmenopausal strategy to maintain bone mass

In Your Fifties

Bone Activity
Menopause usually occurs; sharp drop in estrogen precipitates a two-year postmenopausal surge in bone loss

Diet
Focus on healthy whole foods, such as whole grains, fresh fruits and vegetables, chicken, fish, and lean meats; minimize foods with added fat or sugar

Calcium
1,200–1,500 mg

Lifestyle
Repeat DEXA scan within two years of cessation of menses to determine if bone loss is occurring; maintain regular weight-bearing aerobic and anaerobic exercise program; add flexibility, coordination, and balance exercises to daily regimen; treat any bone loss proactively with medication

In Your Sixties and Beyond

Bone Activity
Bone density subject to lifestyle forces

Diet
Focus on healthy whole foods, such as whole grains, fresh fruits and vegetables, chicken, fish, and lean meats; minimize foods with added fat or sugar

Calcium
1,200–1,500 mg

Lifestyle
Repeat DEXA scan every two years if you have osteopenia or osteoporosis, or every five years if bones are still dense; balanced and varied exercise program is mandatory; attention to diet is important, especially if living alone

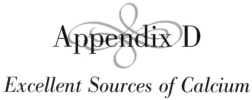

Appendix D

Excellent Sources of Calcium

Check out the list below to supply your bones with food sources that have other valuable nutrients, too. (Vitamin D that is critical to the absorption of calcium is present only in milk.)

Approximately 400 mg calcium per serving
8 oz. yogurt (plain, low-fat, or nonfat)
3 oz. sardines

Approximately 300 mg calcium per serving
1 cup milk (nonfat, low-fat, whole, chocolate, or buttermilk)
1/2 cup ricotta cheese
1 oz. Swiss cheese
1 cup yogurt (fruit-flavored)
1 cup pudding or custard

Approximately 200 mg calcium per serving
1 oz. most cheeses
1 cup ice cream or ice milk
1 cup macaroni and cheese

Approximately 200 mg calcium per serving (*continued*)

3 oz. salmon

1 cup mustard greens

1/2 cup collard greens

1 cup kale

Approximately 100 mg calcium per serving

1/2 cup cottage cheese

8 raw oysters

1/2 cup spinach

1/2 cup bok choy

3 oz. tofu

1 cup raisins (seedless)

1 tbsp blackstrap molasses

1 cup most dried beans and legumes (cooked)

1 tbsp nonfat dry milk

3 oz. shrimp (canned)

1 stalk broccoli

1 cup mushrooms

1 cup dates (chopped)

1/2 cup turnip greens

1 cup most nuts

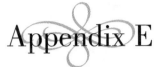

Appendix E

Questions to Ask Your Doctor

A conversation with your doctor about osteoporosis will help you better understand your own risk for the disease and your prospective prevention or treatment options. Here are a number of questions that you can use in discussing osteoporosis with your doctor:

- Based on my medical history, lifestyle, and family background, am I at risk for osteoporosis?
- How do I know if someone in my family suffered from osteoporosis? What physical signs or symptoms should I be looking for?
- Am I currently taking any medication that puts me at higher risk for developing osteoporosis?
- How do I best prevent (or treat) osteoporosis?
- How do I know if my bone density is low?
- How much calcium is right for me?
- How do I best obtain this calcium?
- Should I engage in exercise? What kind of exercise is best? How often should I exercise?
- How do I know if I have fractured a bone in my spine?

If you have osteoporosis or if your doctor believes you are at high risk for the disease, you may want to ask the following questions:

- What medications are available to help me?
- What are the benefits and side effects of these medications?
- Will these medications interact with other medications I am already taking for other conditions?
- How do I know that my prevention or treatment program is effective?
- Do any of the medications I am taking for other conditions cause dizziness, light-headedness, disorientation, or a loss of balance that could lead to a fall?

Appendix F

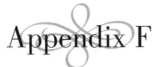

Calcium Supplements and Drug Interactions

When taken together, calcium supplements may interact with some drugs. In some cases the calcium supplement counteracts the absorption or effect of the drug, or the way it is broken down in the body; in others the drug interferes with calcium absorption. These interactions can be avoided when the calcium supplement and the medication are taken two hours apart, or when the supplement is taken two hours before or after a meal with the food.

Drug (generic)	Interaction with calcium
Aspirin	Decreased absorption of aspirin
Barbiturates (phenobarbital, amobarbital)	Decreases absorption of calcium
Bile acid sequestrants used to treat high blood pressure or lower cholesterol (cholestyramine, colestipol, and colesevelam)	Interferes with normal calcium absorption and increases the loss of calcium in the urine
Bisphosphonates (alendronate, risedronate)	Calcium interferes with absorption of bisphosphonates
Corticosteroids	Reduces absorption of calcium

continued on next page

Drug (generic)	Interaction with calcium
Digoxin	High levels of calcium may increase the likelihood of a toxic reaction to digoxin; low levels of calcium cause this medication to be ineffective; blood calcium levels should be monitored closely
Hydrochlorothiazide-based diuretics	Raises calcium levels in the blood to high, potentially damaging to kidneys
Loop-based diuretics (furosemide and bumetanide)	Decreases calcium levels in blood
Potassium-sparing diuretics (Amiloride)	May decrease the amount of calcium excreted in the urine (and subsequently increase calcium levels in the blood), especially in people with kidney stones.
Antibiotics (Gentamicin)	Calcium creates potential for toxic effects of this drug on kidneys
Type 2 diabetes medications (Metformin)	Calcium can prevent depletion of Vitamin B12 levels precipitate by this drug
Some antibiotics, including tetracyclines and quinolones (ciprofloxacin, levofloxacin, norfloxacin, and ofloxacin among others)	Calcium can decrease absorption of the antibiotic
Seizure medications (phenytoin)	Decreases calcium absorption; vitamin D supplement can prevent this

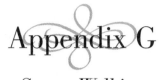

Appendix G

Smart Walking

"The way out is via the door."

—*Lao Tse, Chinese sage*

When it comes to our country's top exercise, we're voting with our feet. More than twenty-two million Americans walk for fitness at least twice a week. Research shows that walking, which has the lowest dropout rate of any fitness activity, can make bones stronger and give you one hour of longevity for every hour you pound the pavement. Start here for a successful fitness program that supports strong bones.

Proper Gear

Shoes

Athletic shoe companies manufacture shoes designed specifically for walking. Ideally, you should invest in a pair of walking or cross-training shoes. If your pace gets very fast, running shoes may be more comfortable. Whatever shoes you decide to buy, make sure they have these characteristics:

- A firm, well-cushioned, flexible sole
- Sturdy uppers made from materials that "breathe"
- Variable lacing options to achieve a custom fit
- Will support your foot for three to six months of daily use (afterward, you can retire them to garden use and invest in another pair)

About the fit of your shoes:

- Since it's not unusual for your feet to swell by one-half size during the day, buy your shoes as late in the day as possible.
- If, like most people, one of your feet is bigger than the other, choose your shoe size based on the larger foot.
- There should be about one-half inch between the end of your longest toe and the front of the shoe.
- The toe box of your shoes should be as wide as possible without allowing the heel to slip. Shoe people use the term "firm heel counter" to describe this feature.
- If you have high-arched feet, you'll need cushioning in your shoes to absorb shock when a forcefully propelled foot hits the ground. If you have a low arch (flat feet), your shoes should have greater support and heel control.

Clothes

If you're walking at a pace sufficient to gain health benefits, you will get hot as you walk. Dress in layers that can be removed as needed. In hot weather, dress to permit circulation of air across your skin. If you walk in cold or rainy weather, choose cotton or wool because its "breathability" will absorb sweat without chilling you. Outdoor recreational stores carry exercise gear made from the newer "breathable" fabrics. These garments combine durability, fashion, and the features that keep you warm and dry, all of which are essential to a satisfactory experience.

Motivational Tools

The average active, nonexercising American walks about three thousand steps a day. Those with a sedentary lifestyle log about one-third that amount. If you want the benefits that fulfill weight-bearing exercise goals and can build strong bones, you need to walk (briskly) at least six thousand steps every day. That fulfills the U.S. Surgeon General's recommendations for physical activity and translates to about three miles. Move through ten thousand brisk paces on most days and you'll lose stored body fat.

A pedometer is a very motivating tool that can track your walking activity. When this small, lightweight tool is calibrated and worn on your waist, it measures the number of steps you take. It reveals, on a minute-to-minute basis, how much exercise you've accomplished and how much you have yet to do. Users discover the fun of knowing how many more steps they take when they use stairs instead of an escalator, or park a car in the outskirts of the mall parking lot, or take that fitness walk every day. A basic pedometer that records steps costs about $35. Additional features that tell time, record distance, and calculate calorie expenditure can double the cost.

A heart rate monitor is the best way to monitor the pace of your workout. This technological marvel has two parts: a transmitter belt that is worn around your chest (under your bra) that picks up the electrical signal your heart delivers when it beats, and a wrist watch that receives the transmitted signal and translates it to heart rate information. You get a continuous, second-to-second, EKG-accurate report of how fast or slow your heart is beating. Heart rate monitors, formerly a piece of equipment only competitive athletes used, are now mainstream. They will bring out the athlete in you. Their cost depends on their features. A monitor that reveals only heart rate is about $60. A sophisticated instrument that has lots of bells and whistles, including the ability to download information into a computer, can run as high as $300.

If you don't like the idea of wearing a strap around your chest, you can buy a MIO® watch, which also reads heart rate but uses different technology. The watch is worn on your left wrist. When you want to know what your heart rate is, you place two fingers of your right hand on special buttons on the watch, and six seconds later you'll know your heart rate. A MIO® watch also tells time and, based on input, records approximate values of calories burned and consumed.

There are more technological exercise marvels being developed every day. Even if you don't fall into the gadget-lover category, surf the Web (try www.rondagates.com first) for these motivational tools that can make the difference between a good walk and a great walk.

Safety

Here are some important safety steps to remember:

- If you've never exercised or have a family history of health problems, check with your doctor regarding your suitability to begin an exercise program.
- Always carry some form of identification with you.
- If you walk alone, let someone know where you're going and when you plan to return.
- Never walk alone in parking garages, stairwells, or less populated areas or at night.
- If you'll be walking for more than thirty minutes, carry a water bottle. Always carry water on a hot day—even when your walk is short.

- Wear reflective clothing when walking at night.
- Vary your route from day to day.
- If your route is along streets without sidewalks, always face oncoming traffic (unless you're on a blind bend). Stay as close as possible to the side of the road.
- Follow all traffic signals—always!
- Be aware of activity around you. Keep an eye out for stray dogs, cars, runners, bicyclists, and suspicious characters.
- If you wear a headphone to listen to a CD or cassette tape, keep the volume low enough that you can hear what's happening around you. Be extra cautious at intersections.

Smart Walking Technique and Training

Technique

Ronda's mentor, Dr. George Sheehan (fondly known as the running doctor), used to give her a lot of static once he heard she led walking classes and taught participants proper walking technique. "Everybody knows how to walk," he said. Then she led him on one of her fitness walks where he was forced to put forth an effort that, for him, was more intensive than his well-integrated and efficient running pace. She shared techniques for fitness walking, to which he responded, "Can you put that down on paper?" This is what she wrote:

- Stand with feet hip-width apart.
- Lift your shoulders, pull them back, then gently press them down.
- Breathe deeply and flatten your bellybutton against your spine as you think about pointing your tailbone toward the ground.

- Pull your chin in and lift your head so your eyes are looking forward.
- Begin to walk, leaning slightly forward from your ankles and bending your arms at your elbows with your palms facing inward.
- Move your arms in opposition to your feet, focusing on the effort that moves your elbows back. As your arm goes forward, it should not go above the bustline or cross in front of your body. If it does, turn your palm up (versus facing your body) as you walk.
- Now focus on your foot roll: Heel strike, roll through the foot, and push off with the forefoot and toes.

Training

Smart Walking uses progressive training techniques. Walking pace is divided into three zones that correspond with the metabolic effects generated by the intensity of the zone:

Level One: Health Zone	16–25 minute mile
Level Two: Fitness Zone	12–16 minute mile
Level Three: Performance Zone	< 12 minute mile

To determine your current level, you will need to go to a track (4 circuits = 1 mile) or measure, by driving, a one-mile distance.

If you can walk one mile, record your time for the walk. If you can't make a mile, figure the time based on the distance you can travel and convert it to a mile. Use the following program to slowly increase your pace. If you are already fit enough to skip the introductory weeks, find the appropriate week that matches your current pace and begin there.

Fifteen-week Smart Walking Program

Use this fifteen-week program as a guide for the duration and frequency of exercise.

Week	1	2	3	4	5	6	7	8
Duration (min.)	10	15	15	20	20	25	25	30
Times (per week)	3	3	4–5	3	4–5	3	4–5	3

Week	9	10	11	12	13	14	15
Duration (min.)	30	35	35	40	40	45	45
Times (per week)	4–5	3	4–5	3	4–5	3	4–5

After fifteen weeks, walk for forty-five minutes three to five times a week to maintain fitness.

Benefits of Smart Walking

The benefits of Smart Walking are physical, emotional, social, and spiritual. They include:

- Improved bone density
- Enhanced aerobic fitness
- Lower blood pressure

- Reduced risk of heart disease
- Lower blood cholesterol
- Increased metabolism
- Decreased body fat (if you reach the Fitness Zone)
- Reduced stress
- Improved sleep patterns and more restful sleep
- Increased lung capacity
- Revitalization

For more on Smart Walking, see "Outwitting Osteoporosis: A Smart Woman's Guide to Smart Walking," a video described in the Resources section.

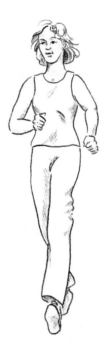

Resources
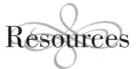

Useful Organizations and Internet Sites

The Internet is a rich resource of information about all aspects of osteo-porosis. Space does not allow us to list all of the useful sites. Arranged in alphabetical order, the following list, which is not comprehensive, includes sites we know are reliable. Remember: as you search for additional infor-mation on and off the Internet, beware of unscrupulous entrepreneurs who may provide you with inaccurate information, myths, and misconceptions about "the silent thief," including some that may use the title of this book. Always look for the names Ronda Gates or Beverly Whipple when you see *Outwitting Osteoporosis*.

American Dietetic Association
www.eatright.org
Promoting optimal nutrition, health, and well-being to consumers through various programs and services is the ADA mission. A referral service to registered dietitians and a resource library with access to an extensive array of databases make ADA a leading source of objective food and nutri-tion information.

American Dietetic Association
216 W. Jackson Blvd.

Chicago, IL 60606-6995
Telephone: 312-899-0040

The American Society for Bone and Mineral Research
www.asbmr.org
ASBMR encourages and promotes the study of bone and mineral metabolism
through annual scientific meetings, an official journal (*Journal of Bone and
Mineral Research*), the *Primer on the Metabolic Bone Diseases and Disorders
of Mineral Metabolism*, and cooperation with other related societies.
ASBMR
2025 M St., NW, Suite 800
Washington, DC 20036-3309
Telephone: 202-367-1161

BreastCancer.org
www.breastcancer.org
Dr. Marisa Weiss, author of *Living Beyond Breast Cancer*, founded a Web
site that helps women make informed decisions about breast cancer. The
site features advice on prevention, treatment, detection, recovery, diagnosis,
and living beyond the disease. It also includes useful information about
osteoporosis. (Internet contact only.)

The Doctor's Guide to the Internet
www.pslgroup.com/osteoporosis.htm
The latest medical news and research information for patients or
friends/parents of patients diagnosed with osteoporosis and osteoporosis-
related disorders. (Internet contact only.)

LIFESTYLES by Ronda Gates

Health Promotion Education

www.rondagates.com

This site, hosted by *Outwitting Osteoporosis* coauthor Ronda Gates, includes updated information about health issues related to exercise, nutrition, weight control, and stress management. There are free fitness tips and free recipes daily. Registration for Gates's complimentary weekly e-mail newsletter will generate a download of low-fat, easy-to-fix recipes.

LIFESTYLES by Ronda Gates

P.O. Box 974

Lake Oswego, OR 97034

Telephone: 503-697-7572

National Dairy Council

www.nationaldairycouncil.org

Have you seen the popular "Got Milk?" mustache advertisements produced by this organization? Perhaps you've seen them at health events where they take your picture—complete with a milk mustache—so you, too, can sell the "drink milk" message. The national organization provides nutrition information through state and regional dairy council units. In addition to using this site, use a search engine to search, for "dairy + council" or "dairy + (your state here)" to find your state organization.

National Dairy Board

National Dairy Council

10255 W. Higgins Rd., Suite 900

Rosemont, IL 60018

National Institutes of Health
Osteoporosis and Related Bone Diseases~National Resource Center
www.osteo.org
NIH ORBD~NRC's mission is to provide patients, health professionals, and the public with important resources and information on osteoporosis and related bone diseases—including fact sheets, research bibliographies, newsletters, links, and print publications.

NIH ORBD~NRC
1232 22nd St., NW
Washington, DC 20037-1292
Telephone: 800-624-BONE
Fax: 202-293-2356

National Osteoporosis Foundation
www.nof.org
The National Osteoporosis Foundation, established in 1986, is a voluntary nonprofit health organization. Its mission is to reduce and ultimately eliminate the widespread prevalence of osteoporosis, through programs of research, education, and advocacy. The foundation's Web site is a rich source of up-to-date factual information about osteoporosis. A $15 membership entitles you to a quarterly newsletter, *Osteoporosis Report*, and seventy-page handbook, *Boning Up on Osteoporosis*. The NOF also manages a database of physicians who specialize in osteoporosis and a database that lists support groups nationwide. If there is no support group in your area, the NOF staff will help you start one.

National Osteoporosis Foundation
1232 22nd St., NW
Washington, DC 20037-1292
Telephone: 202-223-2226
Fax: 202-223-2237

North American Menopause Society

www.menopause.org

This nonprofit membership organization is dedicated to promoting the understanding of menopause and improving the health of women as they approach menopause and beyond. The organization's information is accurate and unbiased. Membership includes a subscription to the newsletter, *Flashes*.

The North American Menopause Society
P.O. Box 94527
Cleveland, OH 44101-4527
Telephone: 440-442-7550
Fax: 440-442-2660

The Osteoporosis Center

www.endocrineweb.com/osteoporosis

This site is an excellent adjunct to *Outwitting Osteoporosis*. Much of the information is the same as that found in the book, but stated in a different way. There are support groups, user forums, and an "unofficial" listing of physicians suggested by site users. (Internet contact only.)

Osteoporosis Society of Canada

www.osteoporosis.ca

This English- and French-language site has extensive news archives, free publications, a bilingual toll-free information line (in Canada only), educational programs, referrals to self-help groups and community resources in Canada, a Calcium Calculator,™ and calcium-enhanced recipes. In addition to its national office, there is a network of affiliate groups in communities throughout Canada.

> Osteoporosis Society of Canada
>
> 33 Laird Dr.
>
> Toronto, Ontario M4G 3S9
>
> Telephone: In Canada: 800-463-6842 (English);
>
> 800-977-1778 (French); in the United States: 416-696-2663
>
> Fax: 416-696-2673

Speaking of Women's Health

www.speakingofwomenshealth.com

We love this organization, and if you have attended a Speaking of Women's Health conference, you know why. Each year the nonprofit foundation manages conferences in more than twenty cities nationwide for the purpose of educating women on how to make informed decisions about their health, well-being, and personal safety. The site lists conference locations, charts the foundation's history, reviews presentations by the prestigious speakers at each event, and provides useful health information for use in your daily life. (Internet contact only.)

The Society for Women's Health Research
www.womens-health.org

The Society for Women's Health Research is the nation's only nonprofit advocacy group whose sole mission is to improve the health of women through research. Since 1990 the Society has fought to increase public and private funding for research on women's health; encourage the study of basic biological and physiological differences between women and men and how those differences affect both health and disease; and promote the appropriate inclusion of women in medical research studies. Many of the studies cited in this book are a result of their efforts.

The Society for Women's Health Research
1828 L St., NW, Suite 625
Washington, DC 20036
Telephone: 202-223-8224
Fax: 202-833-3472

The U.S. National Library of Medicine's
MEDLINEplus® Health Information
www.nlm.nih.gov/medlineplus

MEDLINEplus® is a gold mine of up-to-date, quality health-care information from the world's largest medical library, the National Library of Medicine at the National Institutes of Health. Its experienced staff of information experts reviews hundreds of government and nongovernment publications, brochures, databases, and Web sites in order to link the public with the most reliable and authoritative information. (Internet contact only.)

Books and Videos to Support
Good Eating and Exercise Habits

Books

The Ultimate Fit or Fat
Covert Bailey

Covert Bailey's done it again—he's revised his popular *Fit or Fat*. Though retired from public speaking, Bailey remains at the top of his game as a writer. The title is misleading, though. The book is based on the necessity to address fitness issues from the perspectives of the fit and not so fit. There is a focus in this third edition on weight lifting, which is highly recommended by your authors to strengthen the bones of the upper body and jump-start your metabolism. The book includes a guide, with pictures, for a home strength-building program. Also look for *Fit or Fat* and *The New Fit or Fat* at your library.

Strength Training Past 50
Wayne L. Westcott, Ph.D., Thomas R. Baechle, and Mark Williams

Strength training is an equal-opportunity exercise system. Regardless of how old you are when you start, strength training has nearly immediate benefits: more muscle mass, more strength, and a higher fat-burning metabolism. This book, which has 130 photos, gives older exercisers all the information they need to get started, including advice on testing for strength and how to pick a qualified personal trainer. Fitness expert Wayne Westcott and supporter Tom Baechle present thirty-nine safe and effective exercises as part of a ten-week strength training plan.

We have a problem with the "for Dummies" books, as we don't believe any woman is a dummy. Just close your eyes to get past the title and into the useful information inside the following three books.

Fitness for Dummies
Suzanne Schlosberg and Liz Neporent
This book is a perfect starter for fitness novices interested in general fitness information. You will learn everything you need to know about starting and maintaining a fitness program—getting motivated, choosing a gym, building strength and aerobic endurance, and buying home exercise equipment. These well-known health writers tell it with wit and style.

Workouts for Dummies
Tamilee Webb and Lori Seeger
This book starts with topics as basic as choosing shoes and warming up. Then it covers everything you'll need to create an effective exercise program, starting with an explanation of body types (so you don't think you'll end up looking like Cindy Crawford if you don't already) and the workouts that suit your body type. The book gives directions for stretches, aerobic exercises, muscle conditioning (using weights, furniture, exercise bands, and bars), and workouts for different locations.

Weight Training for Dummies
Suzanne Schlosberg and Liz Neporent

If you want a more strenuous strength-training program using free weights and gym machines, try this book. With plenty of easy-to-understand instructions for beginners, this book also includes information for those who have been training a while. It's pumped up with more than one hundred photos and illustrations of the best exercises for the major and minor muscle groups—exactly what you need for an osteoporosis-prevention workout.

Pedometer Walking
Robert Sweetgall

Robert Sweetgall has walked across the United States seven times, including an unprecedented 11,208-mile walk through all fifty states in 365 consecutive days. This is our favorite of Robert's twelve books on walking and wellness. It includes seventy-eight pages of useful information on how to buy, calibrate, and use a pedometer, followed by a handy logbook designed especially for people who use this terrific tool. (If you can't find it at a bookstore, call Creative Walking, 800-762-9255.)

Nutrition for Women
Elizabeth Somer, M.A., R.D.

This is the best comprehensive nutrition book you can buy. It is highly rated by all book vendors because its advice is written in a clear and approachable style. Somer (who appears regularly on the *Today Show* and *Good Morning America*, and has had a PBS special) reviewed more than two thousand recent studies to prepare this book, which includes information about how to reduce the risk of most disorders, including heart disease, fibromyalgia, cancer, chronic fatigue, and osteoporosis. You'll learn how to lose weight and keep it off, combat fatigue and stress, boost energy, choose the best organic foods and supplements, and look and feel younger. Simple tips on how to prepare tasty, nutritious meals and snacks in minutes is included, as well as how to eat to reduce symptoms of PMS and menopause.

Smart Eating

Ronda Gates and Covert Bailey

This book offers an alternative to dieting, with a revolutionary way to think of food as nutrition. It uses simple guidelines to let you make the food choices that ensure you get the nutrients you need for good osteoporosis prevention and general health (and weight loss). The process is simplified by the Smart Eating "Food Target"—a unique graphic that grades foods according to their fat and fiber content.

Smart Eating is designed for anyone who wants to eat smart—men and women, vegetarians, people with weight problems, athletes, healthy people, and even those with medical problems like osteoporosis and diabetes. It includes two hundred recipes keyed to the Food Target. You'll never diet again. Call 800-863-6000 or visit Ronda's Web site (www.rondagates.com) to order a discounted copy plus a free Smart Eating poster.

Nutrition Nuggets and More

A companion to *Lowfat Lifestyle*

by Ronda Gates

This book is filled with useful information for women of all ages seeking to improve their education about nutrition. In addition to easy-to-read, timeless information about caffeine, salt, sugar, the various fats, supermarket savvy, and restaurant survival, there are ten motivating stories about women who struggled and made lifestyle changes. Call 800-863-6000 or visit Ronda's Web site (www.rondagates.com) to order a copy.

Home Exercise Videos

Outwitting Osteoporosis: A Smart Woman's Guide to Smart Walking
www.rondagates.com

When it comes to walking, certified exercise specialist Linda Warren is the best. She and Ronda Gates, who have collaborated on a number of exercise programs over the years, came up with this video that is a consumer's guide to walking for fitness. This is not a workout. It is everything you need to know before you start a walking program, including correct technique, how to dress and choose shoes, and how to train effectively using the walking guidelines provided in *Outwitting Osteoporosis*. Linda's no-nonsense strategies will help you strengthen bones *and* get fit (and burn fat) fast.

Be Bone Wise™ *Exercise*
National Osteoporosis Foundation Video
www.nof.org

This is the official weight-bearing and strength-training exercise video of the National Osteoporosis Foundation. The five-part video, led by Lisa Hoffman, M.A., includes both muscle-toning and weight-bearing aerobics. It is a forty-one-minute, beginner-level workout with exercises that are gentle and easy to follow.

Better Bones & Balance

www.betterbonesandbalance.com

This forty-five-minute video is an outgrowth of a research study on the effects of long-term exercise participation on bone mass, conducted by Christine Snow, Ph.D., and her associate, Janet Shaw, Ph.D., at the Bone Research Laboratory at Oregon State University. It provides an easy-to-follow routine designed to increase muscle strength and endurance. The progressive program can be performed with or without a weighted vest (beginners start without the vest) that increases the load for exercises, which include resistance training and controlled jumping routines.

Collage Video

www.collagevideo.com

This organization's site offers sixty- to ninety-second previews of the several hundred videos that they stock. They also offer a printed catalog that describes each video, and a toll-free service with telephone representatives who can help you choose the video that matches your needs and fitness level. Call 800-433-6769 or e-mail collage@collagevideo.com for a catalog.

HomeWorkout.com

www.homeworkout.com

There is no catalog for this company and no toll-free consultation service, but they have a slightly different selection of videos, sell books and exercise equipment, and offer profiles of exercise leaders.

Smoking Cessation Programs

Ready, Set, Stop

Registered nurse Fern Carness, a former smoker, has created a four-tape audio series, program worksheets, food and activity planners, and other materials to help smokers stop their smoking habit. Call 800-950-9355.

Smokenders

www.smokenders.com

Smokenders is an educational program having as its goal not only the cessation of smoking but the enjoyment of not smoking and being comfortable as a nonsmoker.

901 N.W. 133rd St., #A

Vancouver, WA 98685

Telephone: 800-828-HELP

Drug Interactions

www.drugstore.com/pharmacy/drugchecker

Find out if your medicines interact by creating a list of products you use, including prescription and nonprescription drugs, herbs, vitamins, and supplements. The site also checks for interactions with alcohol, food, and tobacco.

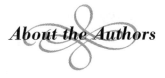

About the Authors

Ronda Gates

Ronda Gates, M.S., is a health promotion educator whose company, LIFESTYLES by Ronda Gates, develops and delivers programs and products to support lifestyle change.

In 1978 Ronda exchanged the white coat she had worn during her seventeen-year career as a hospital pharmacist for a pair of athletic shoes, and never looked back. Her corporate fitness business precipitated graduate health studies, many prestigious awards and fellowships, and a professional career that reflects her effort to make sense of the conflicting information, myths, and misconceptions about women's health.

When Ronda is not on the road lecturing about the many aspects of making healthy lifestyle changes, she is writing about them for publication in the press, magazines, and on the Internet. She maintains her good bone health by teaching a daily dance fitness class and "recreates" in her garden, on a bicycle, and by hiking hills nationwide.

Ronda, the mother of two grown children, Rebecca and Caleb, lives in Lake Oswego, Oregon. You can learn more about her at the LIFESTYLES by Ronda Gates Web site (*www.rondagates.com*). She can be contacted at *ronda@rondagates.com* or 503-697-7572.

Beverly Whipple

Beverly Whipple, Ph.D., R.N., F.A.A.N., is a Professor Emerita at Rutgers University, president of the Society for the Scientific Study of Sexuality (2002–2003), vice-president of the World Association for Sexology (2001–2005), director of the International Society for the Study of Women's Sexual Health (2002–2004), and past president of the American Association of Sex Educators, Counselors, and Therapists. She has devoted her professional life to conducting research, teaching, and speaking nationally and internationally about women's health issues and the sensuality and sexuality of women and couples.

Beverly is the coauthor of the international best-seller, *The G Spot and Other Discoveries about Human Sexuality*. She is often featured in articles in many of your favorite magazines. Beverly's ability to make it easy to understand the sexual subjects that mystify women is only one of her many skills. She enjoys using her understanding of complex research (her doctorate is in neurophysiology) to clarify health issues, so women can learn about themselves and accept and enjoy the mysteries of womanhood. Her sense of humor and matter-of-fact, nonjudgmental style have helped women worldwide to understand and deal with the complexities of their lives and relationships.

Beverly has received numerous awards and fellowships for her research contributions to women's health. She lives in Medford, New Jersey, with her husband, Jim. They have two grown children and five grandchildren. She can be contacted at *bwhipple@pics.com* or 609-953-1937.

For more information about Beverly's perspective on sexual health, visit *www.sexualhealth.com*, and for information about women's health and Beverly's publications, go to *www.nursing.rutgers.edu/people/faculty-detail*.

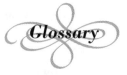

Glossary

17 beta-estradiol patch. Generic name for Estraderm.®

Actonel.® Trade name for risedronate, a bisphosphonate approved by the FDA for the prevention and treatment of postmenopausal osteoporosis, produced by Procter & Gamble Pharmaceuticals and Aventis Pharmaceuticals.

aerobic. Literally means "with oxygen."

aerobic exercise. Exercise that requires oxygen in the muscle to process stored body fat for muscle work. For the purpose of osteoporosis prevention and treatment, this includes walking, jogging, dancing, stair climbing, kickboxing, and other exercise done on the feet on a hard surface.

alendronate. Generic name for the bisphosphonate Fosamax.®

amenorrhea. A lack of menstrual periods.

anaerobic. Literally means "without oxygen."

anaerobic exercise. Exercise that does not require oxygen in the muscle to process energy for muscle work. Strength training, done with weights or elastic bands, is an excellent anaerobic exercise strategy to maintain and build dense bones. It also increases metabolism.

bisphosphonates. A group of drugs that have the ability to attach to calcium in bone and prevent osteoclasts from breaking down the bone.

bone mineral density (BMD). BMD testing measures the density of bones in men and women of all ages.

Calcimar.® Trade name for salmon calcitonin, an injection approved by the FDA for postmenopausal treatment of osteoporosis; produced by Rhone-Poulenc Rorer.

calcitonin. A hormone produced in the thyroid gland that helps regulate calcium metabolism.

calcium. The most important mineral in bone. Calcium plays an essential role in the development and maintenance of a healthy skeleton. If calcium intake is inadequate, calcium is mobilized from the skeleton to maintain normal blood calcium level.

calcium carbonate. A naturally occurring form of calcium commonly used in calcium supplements.

calcium citrate, calcium gluconate, and calcium lactate. Synthetic calcium compounds used in calcium supplements.

compression fracture. A collapsed fracture of a vertebra or bone in the spine.

conjugated estrogen. Generic name for Premarin.®

cortical bone. The dense (hard) outer layer of bone.

corticosteroid. A group of hormonal substances produced in the adrenal gland. The term is also used to describe a group of medicines that duplicates these substances. Cortisone and prednisone are two well-known versions of these drugs.

dual-energy X ray absorptiometry (DXA or DEXA). A diagnostic test used to assess bone density in the spine, hip, or wrist using radiation exposure about one-tenth that of a standard chest X ray. It is the gold standard for measuring the density of bone.

ERT. Estrogen replacement therapy.

Estrace.® Trade name for an oral estrogen, approved by the FDA for the prevention of osteoporosis; produced by Bristol-Myers Squibb.

Estraderm.® Trade name for 17 beta-estradiol patch approved by the FDA for the prevention of osteoporosis; produced by Novartis Pharmaceuticals.

Estratab.® Trade name for esterified estrogen, approved by the FDA for the prevention of osteoporosis; produced by Solvay Pharmaceuticals.

esterified estrogen. Generic name for Estratab.®

estrogen. One of a group of hormones that controls female sexual development.

estrogen replacement therapy (ERT). Administration of the female hormone estrogen; for women who have had a hysterectomy (removal of the uterus).

exercise. An intervention long associated with strong bones. This includes aerobic exercise done on a hard surface and strength-training anaerobic exercise. Coordination, balance, and flexibility exercises improve balance and can prevent falls.

Evista.® Trade name for raloxifene, a selective estrogen receptor modulator (SERM) approved by the FDA for the prevention and treatment of osteoporosis; produced by Eli Lilly & Co.

family history. A risk factor for osteoporosis fractures; defined as a maternal and/or paternal history of hip, wrist, or spine fracture when the parent was age fifty years or older.

FDA. Food and Drug Administration.

fluoride. A compound that stimulates the formation of new bone by enhancing the recruitment and differentiation of osteoblasts. It has not been approved to prevent or treat osteoporosis.

Forteo.® Trade name for the synthetic parathyroid hormone teriparatide, approved by the FDA to treat osteoporosis in men and postmenopausal women who are at high risk for a fracture; produced by Eli Lilly & Co.

Fosamax.® Trade name for alendronate, a bisphosphonate approved by the FDA for the prevention and treatment of postmenopausal osteoporosis; produced by Merck & Co.

fracture. A break in a bone.

hormone replacement therapy (HRT). A general term for all types of estrogen replacement therapy (ERT) when given along with progesterone, either cyclically or continuously. HRT is generally prescribed for women after natural menopause or surgical removal of both ovaries. In October

2002, the NIH and FDA recommended this term be changed to hormone therapy (HT) to more accurately reflect its use.

hormone therapy (HT). A combination of estrogen and progesterone. Used to treat menopausal symptoms and to help maintain bone density.

low bone mass. See osteopenia.

menopause. The completion of the ovarian transition, marked by the last menstrual period. (Menopause is considered complete when a woman has been without menstrual periods for one year.)

Miacalcin.® Trade name for salmon calcitonin, a nasal spray approved by the FDA for postmenopausal treatment of osteoporosis; produced by Sandoz Pharmaceuticals.

normal bone mass. The designation for bone density within one standard deviation of the mean for young normal adults (T-score above –1 SD).

Ogen.® Trade name for piperazine estrone sulfate, approved by the FDA for the prevention of osteoporosis; produced by Upjohn.

ossification. The process by which cartilage is converted to hard bone.

osteoblast. A cell that forms bone.

osteoclast. A cell that breaks down bone.

osteopenia. A condition characterized by a decrease in bone density below normal but not low enough to render a diagnosis of osteoporosis (T-score between –1 and –2.5 SD).

osteoporosis. A chronic, progressive disease characterized by low bone mass and deterioration of bone tissue, leading to bone fragility and an increase in risk of fracture (T-score at or below –2.5 SD).

peak bone mass. The maximum bone mass achieved during skeletal growth, which occurs at young adulthood.

peripheral fractures. Nonvertebral or nonspine fractures, including those of the hip, wrist, forearm, leg, ankle, foot, rib, and sternum.

piperazine estrone sulfate. Generic name for Ogen.®

Premarin.® Trade name for conjugated estrogen, an oral estrogen replacement therapy approved by the FDA for the prevention and management of osteoporosis; produced by Wyeth Ayerst.

prevention of osteoporosis. The practice of preventing bone mineral density from dropping lower than 2.5 standard deviations below the mean for young, normal, adult women; commonly used to describe the prevention of osteoporosis-related fractures.

previous fracture. A risk factor for fractures; defined here as a history of a previous fracture after age forty.

raloxifene. Generic name for the SERM Evista.®

remodeling. An ongoing dual process of bone formation (by osteoblasts) and bone resorption (by osteoclasts) in an adult.

resistance training (strength training). A method of strengthening muscle by increasing the force of contraction of the muscle using weights, elastic bands, or other strategies. This effort, performed consistently, creates a force on bone that increases its density.

resorption. The loss of substance (in this case bone) through physiological or pathological means.

risedronate. Generic name for the bisphosphonate, Actonel.®

risk factors. Factors that increase the risk of an occurrence. Osteoporosis risk factors include low bone mineral density, a genetic predisposition to the disease, excessively low body weight or small frame size, previous fracture, a sedentary lifestyle, and smoking.

SD. Standard deviation.

single-energy X ray absorptiometry (SXA). A diagnostic test used to assess bone density. It is *not* used to measure bone density in the hip or spine, but is useful for peripheral sites.

steroids. A class of synthesized chemical compounds that mimics hormones. They include estrogen, testosterone, cortisone, and prednisone.

standard deviation (SD). A measure of variation of a distribution.

strength training. See resistance training.

SXA. Single-energy X ray absortiometry; used to assess bone density.

testosterone. One of the sex hormones, or androgens, produced in men and women. It encourages the growth of bone and muscle in men.

trabecular bone. The soft, spongelike inner core of bone.

T-score. In describing bone mineral density (BMD), the number of standard deviations above or below the mean for young, normal adults.

ultrasound densitometry. A diagnostic test used to assess bone density at the ankle or knee.

vitamin D. A fat-soluble vitamin useful to prevent and treat osteoporosis.

weight-bearing exercise. Exercise that is done in an upright position, with the feet impacting a hard surface. Some popular weight-bearing exercises are walking, running, stair-stepping, stair climbing, skating, dancing, tennis, and gymnastics.

Z-score. In describing bone mineral density (BMD), the number of standard deviations above or below the mean for women (or men) your age.

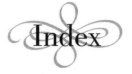

Index

Mesomorphs, 29
Miacalcin, 84, 93
Milk, 34–35, 109, 111
Milk-free diets, 110
Mylanta, 51
Mylicon, 51

National Osteoporosis Foundation, 64,
    102, 143
No-Doz, 42

Ogen, 76
Oophorectomy, 14
Ortho-Est, 76
Orwell, Dr. Eric, 147
Osteoblasts, 15, 19–20, 48
Osteoclasts, 15, 20, 35, 81
Osteopenia, 4, 68–69, 73–94
Osteoporosis. *See also* Prevention;
    Treatment
  BMD scoring, 68–69
  deaths from, xiv, 5, 144
  diagnostic tests for, 64–71, 154
  incidence of, xiv, 4, 143–144
  menopause and, 3, 6, 15–16
  primary vs. secondary, 5–6
  risk of fractures, 4, 52–53,
    70, 144
  statistics on, xiv, 3–4, 143–144
Ovariectomy, 14
Ovaries, 10
Over-exercise, 30, 37, 40, 56
Ovulation, absence of, 56–57

Painful intercourse, 59

Pain treatment, for fractures, 84,
    91–93
Parathyroid gland, 21
Parathyroid hormone, 51, 69, 84–85,
    93, 147
Peirce, Andrea, 89
Perimenopause, 11–15, 59
Phenobarbital, 50
Phenytoin (Dilantin), 50
Physical therapy, 93, 157–158
Phytoestrogens, 89–90
Pilates, 99, 129
Pituitary gland, 10, 20, 46
Postmenopausal zest, 11
Prednisolone, 49
Prednisone, 48, 49
Pregnancy, 15, 55, 57, 157
Premarin, 76
Premphase, 77
Prempro, 77, 78
Prevention
  in children, 15, 20, 155–156
  diet, 107–113
  exercise, 127–136
  lifestyle issues, 137–140
  medications for, 75, 80, 82
  in men, 148
  supplements, 85, 115–125
Primary osteoporosis, 5–6
Progesterone
  absence of ovulation
    and, 57
  in HRT, 75, 76–77, 78
  and menstrual cycle, 10
  and perimenopause, 14

Beyond Words Publishing, Inc.

OUR CORPORATE MISSION
Inspire to Integrity

OUR DECLARED VALUES
We give to all of life as life has given us.
We honor all relationships.
Trust and stewardship are integral to fulfilling dreams.
Collaboration is essential to create miracles.
Creativity and aesthetics nourish the soul.
Unlimited thinking is fundamental.
Living your passion is vital.
Joy and humor open our hearts to growth.
It is important to remind ourselves of love.

To order or to request a catalog, contact
Beyond Words Publishing, Inc.
20827 N.W. Cornell Road, Suite 500
Hillsboro, OR 97124-9808
503-531-8700

You can also visit our Web site at *www.beyondword.com*
or e-mail us at *info@beyondword.com*.